Be
FINE

YOUR DRUG FREE PRESCRIPTION TO AGE WELL, BEAT BULGE, AND STOP DISEASE

DR. LISA LESLIE-WILLIAMS

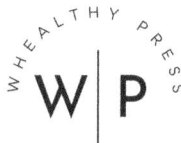

WHEALTHY PRESS

W | P

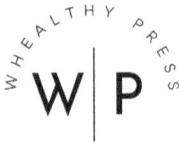

Library of Congress Control Number: 2023907887

ISBN-979-8-9881784-0-8 (hardcover)

ISBN-979-8-9881784-1-5 (paperback)

ISBN-979-8-9881784-2-2 (ebook)

Printed by Whealthy Press, in the United States of America

In memory of my dear friend
Keshema Abramsen-Webbe.
Your memory lives on.

CONTENTS

INTRODUCTION

I wrote this book not just as someone born and rooted in nature, not just as a clinically trained and educated healthcare professional, and not just as a busy home educator, but as a woman who fought her own health battles and won.

I want to teach you how to do the same.

I wrote this book because if I don't tell you these things, I'm not confident that anyone will.

I wrote this book because too many bright, talented people are being sacrificed in a system that's broken, and they are living in bodies that no longer support them. It's time to pivot from a "pill for every ill" to leaning on whole foods to support the healthy living you deserve.

Having the courage to write my own prescriptions for health and wellness led me here. Now I'm ready to take you with me.

This book is organized into four main sections that correspond to the acronym FINE:

F – Focus/Food/Fast
I – Inflammation/Immunity
N – Nutrients
E – Elimination/Exercise/Environment

Are you ready to **Be FINE**? The steps to age well, beat the bulge, and stop disease are on the pages of this book. Do you want it? First you must have a laser focus and be willing to fight for it.

Before I dive into the content, I'd like to properly introduce myself so you can understand my background and why I'm so passionate about helping you on your wellness journey.

I've had my share of wellness lessons. Some people would call them medical emergencies, but it doesn't matter what we call them. What matters is that those experiences helped me, and they can help you too.

Hitting rock bottom for me was not just metaphorical but also physical. Finding myself bruised, battered, bloodied, and broken with my face pressed against a cold bathroom floor was a wake-up call like no other. The learning that took place through that experience and others has allowed me to rid myself and other people of conditions such as micro-nutrient inadequacy, immunodeficiency, joint pain, unwanted weight gain, asthmatic tendencies, skin maladies, cystic ovaries, and low energy, to name a few. The confidence that comes with knowing that true healing comes from the inside out, not the outside in, is seldom taught and is quietly suffocated in exchange for comfort and a reasonable co-pay.

As a clinically trained pharmacist, online content creator, wellness curator, media spokesperson, and homeschooling mom, I didn't think I'd be writing a book about tapping your body's ability to heal and thrive naturally. But it turns out that when properly supported, the body can do just that. Eventually, I figured out what I was trained to do, and I opened my eyes about what I was born to do. I hope you'll join me, but first, here's a look at where it all began.

WHERE IT ALL BEGAN

My path on this wellness journey started in the land of my birth. I'm talking about the lush, tropical island of Dominica, West Indies, regarded globally as one of the places with the most centenarians per capita and once home to the oldest person alive. This is an important aspect of my wellness roots. Its significance did not fully hit me until I was much older.

Also known as the nature island, Dominica has food that is as natural as it comes. Three hundred sixty-five rivers flow freely (enough to visit one every day of the year), and curvaceous mountains burst above the turquoise Caribbean Sea. Dominica is regarded as one of the healthiest places on earth.

In Dominica, my grandparents lived in the countryside, and life was very simple. Like many people of that place and time, my mom's father was a farmer and fisherman who lived off the land. He planted crops, including dasheens, yams, plantains, tanias, and bananas. He grew bay leaves to make bay oil, which he sold commercially. He harvested vanilla and sold vanilla beans. He often took my mom with him to tend to the land while he worked.

My maternal grandmother, who passed away before I was born, planted red peas and pigeon peas. During that time, fruit juice was made rather than bought and was not always readily available. Money was tight, so having bread was a treat, and only eaten on Sundays or major holidays such as Easter and Christmas.

I relished stories my mom shared about feasting on mangoes, pineapples, native almonds, and sea grapes for breakfast and as an after-school snack. In her backyard, beautiful breadfruit, banana, coconut, avocado, cocoa, and coffee trees decorated the fertile ground.

When I was a young girl and wanted a cup of hot chocolate, I drank a cup of cocoa te. There was no powdery mix to scoop from a can and no commercial syrup to add to hot milk. The fresh cocoa beans, after being picked and roasted, had spices added, and then rolled into proper sticks for cocoa tea.

Adults went through a similar arduous effort to get a morning cup of Joe—picking, drying, roasting, and grinding coffee beans before eventually making the perfect cup.

On my father's side of the family, it wasn't abnormal for my grandmother to take long walks in her village. She lived up a steep hill and never owned a car. She walked up and down the hill often to go to the corner store. My paternal grandfather was also a farmer and nurturer of the land.

Freshwater rivers flowed freely, and taking a swim in one of them after a long day was always a welcome treat. In days past, wellness was built into lifestyle, contrary to lifestyle trying to accommodate wellness.

When I was three, my parents moved from Dominica to the U.S. Virgin Islands, America's Caribbean Paradise and my forever island home. When I started school, I became aware that many of my friends ate differently than I did. Soon I was no match for the colorful cereal boxes and catchy jingles that seduced my eyes, ears, and later my palate. I was the new kid who was adjusting to a new island life. I counted it a good day when Mom stopped at the Golden Arches on a Friday evening on her way home from work.

Even so, the Virgin Islands did provide an authentic life in the Caribbean. Tapping into nature for health and healing was a normal way of life for my family. If I came down with a cold, my mom made a homemade concoction of honey, lemon, and herbs, and then rubbed me down with Bay Rum. She rarely gave me a spoonful of store-bought cough syrup first—but did, if she thought she really needed to.

It was customary for locals to seek out the salty, blue-green waters to soothe their aches and pains. The bright, pearly sand made a great natural skin exfoliator steeped in salty nutrients and baked in the island sunshine. I never worried about my vitamin D blood levels or even knew that was something I should keep track of. And I'm pretty sure that in the form of various fruits and vegetables, vitamins A, B, C, and lots of fiber grew in my backyard as well as my neighbors'. Tea didn't often come from a tea bag but from a garden that was easily accessible on any given day.

It's not that I had a perfect childhood. To my mother's chagrin, I didn't always want to eat the right foods. But when you grow up knowing what natural food is, you yield to the centripetal force of home as you get older, and that's how it should be.

At an early age, I was a finger sucker, and I paid dearly for my transgression. The fresh sap from a cut of aloe was my mother's solution. The sap was so bitter that it didn't take long for me to nip that habit in the bud.

When I was around six years old, my parents moved to a new place with a backyard full of fruit trees. It would be our new home for a while. Papayas, mangoes, soursop, cherries, and sugar apples are just some of the fruit trees I remember. I'm sure there were herbs too, but I was more interested in the sweet, delicious fruit. I called our backyard the Garden of Eden.

I grew up with a great respect for nature. Every June, the calm seas could turn into a deadly force of water and howling winds in the form of a hurricane that would sweep homes away and make the Big Bad Wolf look like meek Little Bo Peep. And when I wrote about Hurricane Hugo for a sixth-grade school assignment, I realized I had a knack for creative writing. Mr. Newton, the school principal, hung my paper inside a glass case by the front office so everyone in the school could see it.

Hurricane Hugo not only made me realize my aptitude for writing but was a lesson in gratitude. The powerful storm ripped away our house, rendering us homeless and forcing us to abandon our belongings and seek shelter with just the clothes on our backs. While we were huddled in a nearby church, I saw a glass sliding door blow out like a piece of soft bubble gum. I was eleven years old, and any evidence that I was once a wide-eyed, curly-fro'd baby with my stuffed animals I liked to collect was "gone with the wind."

Written words became my form of expression. I didn't want to become an English teacher, but my Hurricane Hugo paper pinned outside the principal's office gave me a sense of pride and quite honestly piqued my curiosity.

It was also during those elementary years that I developed an appreciation for the health sciences. Everything about how the body operates fascinated me.

Part of my childhood was spent watching a colorful mix of episodes of the geeky children's science show *Mr. Wizard's World*, interspersed with televised beauty pageants, a dose of *Looney Tunes, The Martha Stewart Show,* and a myriad of cooking shows.

In my dreams, I imagined having my own cooking or lifestyle show. But I also had a heart for science and an upbringing steeped in practicality. In my twenties, I got a job as a pharmacy technician at a retail pharmacy. Fielding questions from customers was a great lesson in natural health since many islanders seemed more interested in natural and over-the-counter remedies than the pharmaceuticals their doctors prescribed.

After that introduction to the pharmaceutical industry, I decided to officially hang my hat in the health sciences field. Finishing a bachelor of science degree and later moving on to earn a doctorate in pharmacy, my goal was to help people live healthier, more vibrant lives.

While I was in pharmacy school, an elective class called Complementary and Alternative Medicine caught my attention. The mere idea that holistic medicine is called "alternative medicine" when it has existed since prehistoric times and modern medicine has only been around for about two centuries should make you raise an eyebrow.

After I completed the class, I yearned for more of the same. But modern medicine is far from homeopathic. So I quieted that calling, got a job in retail pharmacy, and did what I was trained and paid well to do. During that time, I saw customers' initial prescriptions slowly turn from one, into three and then into six as the medications created side effects that also needed to be treated.

Eventually, I chose to pivot from my life in retail to focus on a growing family and my passion-led business. What happened next shook me to the core. It reminded me that wellness is not manufactured but a series of daily, calculated steps taken in the direction of a healthier and more energetic tomorrow. It took me back to the core values of using food as medicine and nature to heal. Essentially, I was unlearning and relearning how to take care of God's gift, the body. The body is so intuitively designed that when given the right fuel, tools, and environment, it will exemplify strength, agility, and vitality well into the golden years.

A "lifestyle and nature first" approach helped rid my body of signs of autoimmunity, hormonal imbalance, hair loss, a weakened immune system, and a health fragility I didn't recognize as my own. When my health team couldn't save me, I dove deep out of necessity to relearn, heal, and feel "normal" again.

It may surprise you to know that a typical American spends an average of $1,200 per year on prescription drugs! Even so, the US healthcare system is not even in the top ten global rankings for health. Something is devastatingly wrong, and I started to discover why along the way.

I soon realized that unless you get to the source of what ails the body, the problem continues to perpetuate, and the aftermath is never pretty.

FOCUS, FOOD, FAST

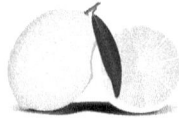

Chapter 1

FOCUS OR FALL

Learn how to break, or prepare to be broken.

Broken.

There comes a time when you have to shift or you'll be shifted. For me, one of those times came before dawn on February 14, 2018.

Yep, you read that right—Valentine's Day.

But before we get to my life-changing morning, let me backtrack a bit. I had been feeling an internal shift for a while, like I was supposed to change my focus.

Three weeks earlier, on January 24, 2018, I had written these words in a post on my blog: "I'm ready for something different. The signs are everywhere, and it's time to change things up. I'm not ready to say in what way or ways yet, but the tides are changing. Things are shifting."

In the early hours of Valentine's Day, I found myself pulling my bruised and bloodied body out of the shower stall. Somehow, after waking up in the middle of the night to use the bathroom, I had lost consciousness.

Bloodied.

Aching.

Convinced it was a dream, I blinked several times, hoping I would wake up. The pain radiating from my lower jaw was undeniable. As I ran my tongue over my teeth, the seriousness of what had just occurred hit me. I felt a jagged, pointed edge that had not been there before.

As startled as I was, I realized I couldn't lie on the cold tiles forever. I hoped I was having a vivid dream, the kind where it feels freakishly real but eventually you wake up. There was blood on the shower stall, and I knew it was my own. My groom was on a business trip, and I would have to get through whatever this was on my own.

I now affectionately call this part of the story "My Bloody Valentine."

I carefully stood up and looked in the mirror. There was a streak of dried blood on my face that led from my mouth to my ear and then to my hairline. The narrow curvature of my chin was now a deep purple hue, and it hurt even to force a smile.

Some of the beautiful white teeth I had flashed in pageants, modeling shows, TV appearances, and photos with my beloved family and friends were now broken.

Red, jagged, broken.

Broken was how my body felt in the wake of what I learned were micronutrient deficiencies, likely stemming from unrecognized nutritional neglect and unintentional lifestyle abuse. After a medical scare a few years earlier, I had removed some potential trigger foods but had unrealized residual damage that was now coming to the surface.

I was also working.

I was working *hard*—homeschooling my two young kids, building an online business, and managing a crazy family travel schedule, all with the love and support of my hard-working groom who traveled extensively for work.

I was exhausted. According to "Dr. Google," I may have experienced an episode of *micturition syncope*.

My web query revealed this: "Micturition syncope or post micturition syncope is the name given to the human phenomenon of fainting shortly after urination. The underlying cause is not fully understood, but it may be a result of vasovagal response, postural hypotension, or a combination thereof."

Basically, it's a phenomenon that could be caused by *anything*.

Google can say what it wants, but truthfully, I was stubborn—successfully stubborn at that. And sometimes the only way to get a stubborn, headstrong, ambitious person like me to slow down and listen is to *take her down*.

As I stared at my damaged face in the mirror, I continued my internal dialogue.

"Am I in the middle of a bad dream? Should I wake the kids?" They were four and seven years old at the time.

"Should I go to the hospital? If I go to the hospital, who will watch the kids in the wee morning hours? Do I have to take them with me? Would such an experience scar them for life?"

Surely I didn't want to startle anyone. I decided to clean up the blood on my face and go back to bed. The faster I could do that, the faster the bad dream would be over—or at least so I thought. It was just after 3:00 a.m., and the sun hadn't risen yet. I was hoping and praying that in the morning I would wake up from the nightmare.

But just in case I wasn't dreaming, I texted a good friend and my groom so they knew what had transpired. Then I went back to sleep.

The scene, I later realized, was eerily similar to an accident I had had on a hot September island day when I was ten years old. I had fallen off my top bunk during the night while trying to share the bed with too many stuffed animals. I banged the side of my head on the corner of a dresser. That was before guardrails were a safety thing. Thank goodness for innovation!

But this time I wasn't a child, and it was different. This time I wasn't trying to hide a gash at the side of my head from my school friends. I was trying to hide my mouth and teeth from my kids. Walking into their room was the hardest part.

Hands over my mouth, I simply said, "While you were sleeping, mommy had an accident. When I remove my hands from my face you will see that it looks different. Don't be scared. It won't be exactly the same. Some of my teeth are a little broken. I'm okay."

Waiting for their approval, I slowly moved my hands to reveal the "brokenness" underneath. Suddenly, their strong, do-it-yourself momma didn't seem so strong anymore. The accident left me pretty shaken up.

On the advice of a friend, later that day, I frantically scribbled my thoughts about the accident on the first page of a small gold notebook I had gotten a few years before.

> Woke up overnight twice to use the bathroom. The second time, things didn't go well. Once I came to, it was 3:23 a.m. in the morning. Blood on my towel. Blood in the shower stall, blood on my face. Apparently, I fainted. I don't know why. When I was

about to rise from the toilet, I distinctly remember thinking, "I feel hot." Then after that, my first memory is dragging myself outside the shower stall. My two front teeth got banged up pretty badly. My lower jaw took some blows. But the dentist was able to see me today and fix up my teeth.

It's going to cost me exactly $1,404 for those teeth. B is out of town, and so life goes on. Aunt Flo came today, and I wonder if that had anything to do with it?

Lord, thank you for protecting me. Thanks for healing. Thanks for putting people in my life who love and care for me. My jaw is hurting and bruised, but things will get better. Lord, if you wanted to wake me up . . . I'm listening. I hear you loud and clear. And that's exactly when the *shift* happened.

SHIFT AFFIRMATION

They don't have to like what you say. They don't have to like what you do or how you do it.

Shift happens.

Approval doesn't change purpose or drive when your energy is tapped from a higher source. When your purpose is higher than self, no external forces can throttle that.

Shift happens.

Do you want better health? Go get it!

Do you want to run like you did when you were in college? Go get it! Do you want to live an energetic, abundant life that will make your younger self jealous? Go get it! It's your life.

Shift happens.

Are you tired? Sick and tired? Then you have to *shift*. You want it? Go get it!

But it can only happen if you're willing to get uncomfortable. It can only happen if you're willing to have them talk behind your back.

If everyone is doing it, that's probably not the way to get it done.

It can only happen if you're willing to Fall . . . Fail . . . Unlearn . . . Relearn . . . Blaze a trail . . . Be broken . . . Be rebuilt.

Shift happens.

Potential . . . don't die with it.

Wellness . . . it happens 24/7/365.

Drive . . . it's internal.
Write your own script for health and wellness.
Shift happens.
What's going to be your external *shift*?

YOUR BODY GIVES YOU LIFESAVING SIGNS

Everyone's talking about living their best healthy life these days, but most people don't know where to start. And how do you go about living that life when you haven't been taught how to bring your best healthy version of you into it?

It most likely started a while ago—that on-and-off, nagging health problem you've been trying to resolve—that toxic environment you know you should leave—the daily habits that take you farther and farther away from the health and wellness you ought to have. It started long before you took notice. You were busy living your life, and then *bam!* Now you have no choice but to hit the pause button. You may think it started a few months ago, but your body has overcompensated for so long that you don't even know when it began.

It's smart, you know—your body.

It'll hide imbalance and illness so effectively that you won't even know it's there until the crescendo. You can get your hair done, never miss a manicure, and edit the best pictures and post them on social media while underneath it all, the storm is brewing.

You won't realize it until you go on a much-needed family trip, and as soon as you check into the hotel, you start puking your guts out. You'll think it's a stomach bug until you realize that no one else is getting sick. At that point, you have to take notice. Well, hopefully that doesn't happen to you, but I know firsthand because that's exactly what happened to me one Father's Day.

I didn't see the signs, but three years before "My Bloody Valentine," the first glaring signs were there. But when you're surrounded by other hard-working moms plagued by low energy, skin conditions, cystic ovaries, and digestive issues, it normalizes the cries of unhealthy bodily dysfunction. On top of all that, constantly catching the latest bug from our school-aged kids adds even more logs to the fire.

Maybe your signs look different. Maybe they're migraines, fibroids, chronic fatigue, mental fog, recurrent yeast infections, or that belly bulge that just won't go away.

For me, there was wrenching pain, frequent vomiting, and an emerging dime-sized bald spot. I found the spot when I was combing my hair one day. I went to a few doctors, but the answers were few. They bounced me around like a ping-pong ball, and by the time I got to doctor number three, I knew I had to jump in and take control.

It's then that I made the decision to drive myself to health and recovery. Do you need to do the same?

Modern medicine was failing me, and since I'd seen it happen before to friends, family members, and patients, the signs were easy to recognize.

Having the best insurance can't help if you refuse to put in the necessary work to save yourself. A co-pay is an illusion to better health. It is not the perceived gateway to the unabridged health solutions you seek. Instead, it's a narrow road that directs you toward a preselected path with a mirage of choice. You can see the best-chosen providers, feel good about your co-pay, and still be broken in wellness.

I read other stories online about how it took some people as many as twelve doctor visits to receive a proper diagnosis. I was convinced that rather than continuing to seek a diagnosis, I needed a *wellness awakening*.

MY WELLNESS AWAKENING

Diagnoses can be great tools, but a diagnosis only reveals what's wrong with you. Instead, you should really be focusing on what's wrong with your food, your environment, your habits, and your lifestyle. It's a small shift in thought. It shifts the energy from that of a victim to one of a victor.

So when the well-meaning gastroenterologist mentioned the idea of giving me a "routine" esophagogastroduodenoscopy (EGD), which essentially meant she would shove a camera down my throat to get a better look, I decided I preferred to have cameras *on* me and not *inside* me, and that was the end of playing doctor roulette.

I had the needed mindset shift and decided that whatever I needed to "nurse myself back to health" was what I would seek and soon discover.

I wasn't sure if any of this would work, but I would surely give it a good try. Diagnosis codes are great for insurance billing but not so great for empowerment building. Just because a doctor uses a code doesn't mean you're getting to the root cause. I didn't want to be a long-term patient or a victim of my circumstance. I wanted a *solution*.

If I inadvertently told the wrong person about the task I had assigned myself, they would verbally whip me into guilty submission and advise me to "do the right thing." The right thing in health is what makes those around you feel most comfortable and secure.

"At least take the medicine," one friend told me. "That way you'll at least feel better while you're home with the kids." She was well intentioned, and she was kind of right. The medicine would patch me up on the outside and placate my symptoms.

But would I actually be healthier? I wasn't convinced. It would be like taking a pain reliever for a broken foot, saying the pain was gone but never addressing the fact that your bone was still broken and needed proper mending.

One week after embarking on this solo journey to healing, 50 percent of the symptoms were gone. My skin cleared, the pain stopped, and the vomiting ceased.

A week later, the majority of symptoms I had been experiencing for almost a year were gone. One month later, the emerging dime-sized bald spot I had seen just months before started to fill back in.

In that one month, I was able to rid my body of several unhealthy conditions. Those were the kind of results that were worthy of a cover and front-page headline on any glossy magazine. The headline would read, "Could This Be the Next Breakthrough Drug?" I could see it already.

Four weeks after I implemented my changes, all my outward symptoms were gone. But I wasn't taking a new breakthrough drug. This wasn't even something I had learned as a lifelong student of health or from a formal postgraduate education. It was a change in lifestyle habits—what I ate, how I ate, and when I ate—that gave my body what it needed. It got me on a path to recovery and returned me to the life and health I had known.

I became a normal, healthy human being. Of course, once a year I'd get a stomach bug or some other germ that was running around, but overall, I felt really good. My immunity was good, but I knew it could be better. I had made many changes to my health and my family's health, and wellness came out on top.

My life was not perfect. Although I had been practicing as a licensed healthcare professional, I had lost some of the spark for my innate lifestyle-first approach to wellness. I had first realized that spark in elementary school when teachers used to roll the school's solitary projector in and out of classrooms to show young minds how the human body worked.

I was finding my way back to that passion. I had already pivoted from patent medicine and was now trying to make a name for myself writing and posting content online. I wanted to teach people how to be health-empowered, grab hold of the reins, and take care of their health and wellness as I had learned to do. I was preparing to make a change in focus but was scared to turn the wheel.

So I made some changes—lots of changes. But removal without restoration is an incomplete path to healing. So I had to be taught . . . *again*.

DR. LISA'S NOTES

» Your body seldom throws a tantrum without giving warning signs. What are the glaring warning signs for you?
» See the *shift*, and use it to guide you on a path toward wellness and healing.

WELLNESS PRESCRIPTION

» Identify a recurring warning sign that your body is conveying to you. Be clear, and be specific.
» How has that warning sign negatively affected your life up to this point?

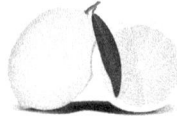

Chapter 2

FOCUS YOUR MIND

Just a slight mindset shift can change the way you think about yourself, your body, and your wellness journey. This slight shift will give you all the power.

Once you've been broken and can feel the shift, it's time to focus.

A problem ensues when you try to shift, primarily because someone tells you to and not because you desire the change for yourself. In those types of situations, behavior modifications don't last.

It's scary to pivot.

That pivot, however, can elicit lifelong transformative change and have a huge impact on your life and the lives of others around you. It's the one thing that can really move the needle.

Thankfully, God pushed me to my breakthrough, and I'd like to help you get to yours too. Here are some helpful thoughts to ponder.

"Everything is created twice, first in the mind and then in reality." —Robin Sharma

"Mind over matter." —Sir Charles Lyell

"If you don't believe it, you won't achieve it." —Traditional saying

There's a reason that sayings like these exist. If you want to get things done, you first have to focus your mind.

The truth is that before you get deeper into this book or start flipping ahead looking for recipes, you have to *get your mind right*. Before you start peeling back the layers of how you need to get your health in order, you first have to get your mind right.

So you want to Be FINE, huh? You can get there.

This is not about fitting into a slinky dress, your favorite t-shirt or skinny jeans. Although that could happen, those reasons don't typically translate into long-term lifestyle habits that last.

Here's why.

Whether you know it or not, we all come into this world with a certain inherited health mindset. From the time we take our first swallow of milk to our dying meal, we all have a mindset when it comes to food. We've heard messages like these: "You need to eat breakfast in the morning." "If you don't eat all your vegetables, you won't get dessert." Maybe you've heard your mom say, "You're a picky eater like your uncle." All these words send messages about health and food.

"You need to eat breakfast in the morning" promotes the mindset that no matter how you feel, breakfast is a necessary part of every day.

"If you don't eat your vegetables, you won't get dessert" sends the message that if you endure this thing that is *bad*, you'll get something *good* in exchange. In other words, vegetables are bad; dessert is good.

Even comparing your eating habits to your uncle's can give you a sense of pride. Maybe you think your uncle is a cool guy and that being compared to him is an honor.

Those food messages strengthen with each exposure and each passing day. Food mindset is often difficult to break or change because it's wrapped deeply in memories. It's steeped in tradition, societal norms, culture, family history, relationships, and conditioning.

That's why you should know that the first step in taking control of your health is to *focus your mind.*

If you don't do that, you're setting yourself up for failure after failure. To take charge of your life, you must be willing to reexamine childhood messages about health and food, and break old habits. Just because you've always done something a certain way doesn't mean you've been doing it the best way for you. Just because your mom always served your meals a certain way doesn't mean she had an exclusive insight into truth.

I know that's hard to hear.

Be willing to break free from the toxic traps that can come with blind devotion to tradition. Doing that will open the door to true health and wellness.

One of the worst things you can do is jump into Be FINE before wrapping your mind around the life change and what it entails. If you don't do that, you will be setting yourself up for failure. Here's why.

YOUR DIETARY JOURNEY

Sometime between the thirteenth and fifteenth week of your mother's pregnancy, you started developing taste buds. The very amniotic fluid in which you lived was flavored with last night's Chinese food, the freshest fruits and vegetables from a bountiful salad, or the rocky road ice cream she craved as a welcome breakfast treat.

You tasted it.

You were enveloped in it.

You bathed in it.

You *liked* it.

You had no say in the matter. She ate what she craved and what she could keep down, hopefully along with some recommended vitamins to keep both of you healthy.

A few months later, you were born. Whether you were breastfed or formula fed wasn't your choice. You ate what you got. Your mom did the best she could. If you were breastfed, your food was flavored by everything mom ate. Whether it was healthy or not, you tasted it. You enjoyed it. You had no choice.

Milkshakes . . . you had them. Steamed kale . . . maybe not so much.

If you were formula fed, you got used to certain flavors as well. Preservatives, soy, and high fructose found their way in there too. By the time you grew teeth and were ready to eat your first real bite, you had a preference. But all was not lost yet.

Your mom read in an article that spinach was good for babies, so she fed you some. You spit it out because you naturally preferred foods such as bananas, carrots, sweet peas, and applesauce. Your mom was tired of "fighting with a baby" and was greatly sleep deprived, so she fed you more of what you liked. Hardly anyone in the house ate spinach anyway. Mom affectionately commented in your presence, "You're just like your daddy— he doesn't like vegetables either." There was comfort in knowing that. So the next time someone dared to overstep your taste bud boundaries, you wrapped those words around you like armor.

Over the next few years, your parents offered you vegetables with little to no expectation that you'd eat them. Perhaps they hid them under a mountain of cheese or submerged them in a lake of ranch dressing.

Every meal, snack, and beverage was purchased and chosen for you. You got your first taste of cake at the age of one, but before that, processed baby foods were a regular staple. At four, your mom took you to preschool and packed the things you liked because she wanted you to eat and not be hungry for the few short hours she was away. After all, food was love, and she was doing her best.

Unbeknownst to you, even the so-called "all natural" and "healthy" snacks were filled with sugar and preservatives. (White flour, sugar, and corn syrup are all "natural" ingredients!) When you were at home, it was more of the same. When you were "good," someone rewarded you with your favorite sweet treat.

If the family had a long, tiring week, everyone went for ice cream. Life was busy, so food delivery offered convenience. Grandma gave you a dollar every week so you could buy yourself a treat. Your unhealthy yearnings were reinforced after every scraped knee, every win, every loss, every heartache, and every heartbreak. Soon, you learned to rely on calorie-dense, nutrient-poor food as a way to cope.

But it wasn't just your family. The restaurant industry knew what kids liked, so the majority of kids' menus had everything you wanted without even asking. Kids ate free with every adult purchase as long as they had refined carbohydrates, entrees cocooned in sugar and the regular dose of artificial colors, flavors, and preservatives.

You may have tried to deviate like my then-five-year-old daughter did at a restaurant when she ordered a kale salad topped with lean protein. The server turned and asked, "Really? Should I give it to her?" A question like that can tumble a child's confidence since the unspoken expectation from adults is *kids don't eat greens or vegetables.*

You couldn't drive until you were sixteen. You didn't pay any bills yet either. So your parents bought the food, and you ate it. Your mom remarked to friends that kids don't like green, leafy vegetables and seem to live on macaroni and cheese, pizza, nuggets, and French fries. Her friends nodded in agreement and said, "It must be something about this younger generation."

By the time you went out to live on your own, you repeated what you'd unknowingly been taught. You started college and could eat whatever you wanted, whenever you wanted. Pizza and energy drinks became your way of life. The occasional fresh, dark green vegetable was out of the picture . . . unless you were one of the fortunate ones.

On the way to class, you grabbed fancy coffees with extra pumps of syrup. It was the only way you could keep up your energy. Your childhood eczema flared under the pressure of exams, and you confidently told the doctor that skin conditions had been your plight since you were a baby.

No one connected your mom's dietary decisions to your skin afflictions; after all, it ran on your dad's side of the family. Both your brothers and your sister had it. You filled your prescription and met your friends for dinner and drinks.

When you hit your thirties, other problems started to pop up that you could no longer ignore—high blood pressure, fibroids, pre-diabetes, difficult periods, diabetes, achy joints, thyroid issues, hormone fluctuations, and digestive issues. And for some reason, those skin flare-ups never really went away. Your doctor started threatening you with words such as *insulin*, *lifestyle changes*, and *exercise*. At that point, you had endured thirty or more years of food conditioning.

You grabbed the new best-selling book with the celebrity TV doctor on the cover. You skimmed through it and tried eating "healthy" foods, but it was difficult because you didn't like them. And the food was so expensive—or at least that was your perception.

"If I'm going to spend that much money on something," you told yourself, "I might as well enjoy it!"

You equated being healthy with deprivation, and you didn't like being deprived. Your job, spouse, and kids were stressful enough. At the end of a long day or week, you *deserved* to eat what you wanted, when you wanted. You ate for recreation, long after your stomach was full.

As a matter of fact, right after the kids went to bed, you went to the freezer and retrieved the double-stuffed cookies from the frozen vegetable bag. *They'll never find them in there!*

You told yourself that when the kids grew up, it would be time to take care of yourself. Almost overnight, they grew up, and you wondered where the time went.

TIME TO CHANGE

Today, it's reinvention time. Now you're investing your time and energy in house renovations, a new business, and volunteerism. But you're always so tired. You grab some eats from your favorite fast-food spot on the way home. That new reality show, *Girrllll… You're Way Too Busy,* is so good. You plan to catch up on the last two seasons after the evening news.

Sound familiar?

That is why lifestyle changes are so challenging. You just can't work on them without some mental logistics built in. You're working on rewiring and reconditioning programming that started even before your parents laid eyes on you. You've been conditioned at every single meal on every single day for twenty, forty, or even more years. Your loved ones have the same thoughts about health and food that you have grown to accept. When you share thoughts and ideas that are contrary, they call you a "health nut."

That's why diets and lifestyle changes don't work without the first step. You have to *focus your mind.*

Sometimes those mindset shifts are hard to achieve due to *cognitive dissonance*—when there is mental stress caused by two opposing beliefs or cognitions that are often contrary to each other.

It's especially challenging when you have been taught or have come to this belief through many years of upbringing and conditioning. Oftentimes, we continue engaging in harmful behavior even if deep down inside we're now in tune with the truth.

And when it comes to making those lifestyle changes around family and friends, you can see why harmful food habits are so difficult to break. You can literally be biting into a cake (made with leftover Halloween candy), knowing it's self-sabotage, and go for another slice. In this case, there is no moderation.

As a society, we would never ask people in addiction recovery to exercise moderation with alcohol, illicit drugs, or nicotine. You either use those things or you don't. But somehow, food addiction gets a free pass. Whether that addiction is to sugar, bread, or rice, it really doesn't matter.

The biggest problem with moderation is that not everyone knows how to moderate.

You literally have to unlearn what you've learned and start over. If you believe that food should be a reward, you will feel deprived when you don't get what you want. If you equate fatty and sugary foods with love, you will feel unloved when the calories stop their never-ending flow.

If certain types of meals bring you comfort, then a major lifestyle change can make you feel vulnerable. If you bond with your friends over food and drinks, you may feel lonely when you change your eating habits and those invitations stop coming. And after that is all said and done, it's hard to be committed to the changes you made.

You'll tell your friends that the plan didn't work because you don't see a correlation. They'll echo your sentiments because if you change, that will challenge them to change too, and they're not ready to change.

The truth is that if you change your mindset, you can change your life. But first, you literally have to unlearn what you've learned about food, about health, and about the role you play in the whole thing. It's not just about mindset. It's about focus.

IT'S ALL ABOUT YOUR FOCUS

It's your health and your responsibility. Shifting the blame won't change the fact that it's time to commit.

Your focus has to be laser sharp, and it has to be adjusted when it gets off track. It has to be unrelenting. You need focus in order to go from "sick and tired" to "pivoting and thriving." If you thought this was going to be a magic pill, it's not. If you thought it would be all warm and fuzzy, that's a lie. But this book will get you from where you are now to where you need to be, and you'll be a HIT (Healthy, Inspired, and Thriving) while you get FINE.

Getting FINE is not just about increasing your lifespan; it's about increasing your *healthspan*. After all, you could live to be eighty-four years old and spend your final thirty years with limited mobility and lack of independence. You could be on so many prescriptions that you resort to carrying them in a plastic grocery bag when it's time for your refills.

The number of years you are independent and active is the key. Being able to show your best moves in the *Soul Train* line is a better indicator of wellness than chronological age. It's not about the number of years you have but the amount of vitality in those years. Similarly, it's not about *when* you start but the fact that you get started.

Research shows that fewer than one in ten people actually keep New Year's resolutions. That's a glaring sign that behavioral change has more to do with mindset than you may think. It's not enough to want something. If you're going to change your behavior, you have to change your mindset.

Here are some thought starters to help you get on the path to being and living mindfully well.

- Every day is a new day.
- The changes I seek can be accomplished every day of the year.
- It's not a diet; it's a lifestyle.
- Exercise is not a chore; it's a privilege.
- Wellness is not a trend; it's an energetic state of being.
- I'm not depriving myself; I'm liberating myself from lifelong disease and illness.

Don't get stuck on simple decisions such as the best time of day to exercise. Instead think of how your body will continue to weaken, how anxiety will tighten its grip, and how illness will ensue if you sit on the couch one more day.

Inaction is a disease of mindset.

So change your mindset, and you can—and will —change your life!

DR. LISA'S NOTES

» The first step to getting FINE is a mindset shift.
» To truly shift, you have to unlearn and relearn your relationship with food.
» Change your mindset; change your life.

WELLNESS PRESCRIPTION

» What is one food or lifestyle habit you need to change? Say it out loud. Call it by its name. Shift the momentum in your favor, and then commit to making one behavioral change today.

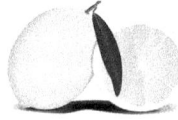

Chapter 3

FOCUS ON YOUR WELLNESS WHY

*It's not about how you feel now. It's about why
you're doing it and how you want to feel later.*

It's more than just saying, "It's the thought that counts." You have to know the "why" behind those thoughts. Identifying your *wellness why* will allow you to move with purpose and conviction. Your *wellness why* will keep you motivated long after the wedding, long after the family reunion, long after the milestone birthday, long after other changes in your life. In fact, the concept of *why* is so important that you'd be hard pressed to start any quality program without it.

The idea of *why* was repopularized with Simon Sinek and other self-help authors. Starting with *why* explains the purpose behind an action. It taps into the part of the brain that connects emotion with behavior. And if that *why* is not compelling enough, guess what? Your wellness dreams will be no more stable than a bowling ball placed on a house built from a deck of playing cards.

Ask yourself this: Why do I want this?

Seriously.

Why do you want to throw all caution to the wind and start making these life-altering decisions? Is it because you want to show up to your class reunion looking fabulous? Are you hoping to snag a date, or are you getting ready to go on vacation?

Is it because you want to show your ex what they're missing out on? Maybe you have a wedding coming up and you're hoping to fit into a dress.

Well, here's the thing: those reasons are not deep enough. They're superficial goals that just don't go the distance. If you want to win and if you really want to go farther, then coming up with your *wellness why* will be challenging. It has to transcend "I want to lose ten pounds before my birthday." Your *wellness why* has to be long-term, and it requires consistent, enduring action in order to sustain success.

HOW I FOUND MY WELLNESS WHY

Some years ago, I found myself on my couch unable to move. I was having the most awful lower stomach pains, and I didn't know why. It was Labor Day, and my groom was in our backyard barbecuing and had absolutely no clue I was suffering or in pain. That wasn't the first time this pain had gripped me, but this time it was hard to ignore or tolerate. Typically, the pain was accompanied by bouts of cyclic vomiting. Some months I was fine, and other months I was down for the count.

One of my lowest points was hurrying the kids into bed before the sun had completely set so I could hurl my face over a cold, porcelain toilet seat. I threw up so much that eventually it became a dry heave.

I felt like an incapable mom. I was eight months into this mystery illness, and already it was hard to cope. I imagined months turning into years, not being able to tuck my kids into bed at night, missing games and events, and not being the type of mom I wanted to be. I thought about friends going through worse things than I was at that time. Seeing them seek treatments, navigate numerous surgeries, and live with recurring illnesses was hard. Truthfully, I feared that would soon be my fate. So at some point, I decided I had had enough.

I didn't have a diagnosis, but I imagined what it could be. I had a friend stricken with cancer, and I knew that life was extremely hard for her and her family. I had numerous friends who suffered from other illnesses such as seizures and migraines of unknown origin, and the answers were few. I thought about other mom friends who were having their own health trials and tribulations.

I didn't want life to be that way.

What if this was my wake-up call? What if this was my opportunity to turn everything around and do health even better than I had been? Before these episodes started, I'd say I was quite healthy. At least I conformed to my concept of what that was at the time. But something was happening, and it shook my body to the core. Right then and there, I knew I had to do more.

Of course, there is always some initial inconvenience with any new life change. But once you realize that the ramifications of any short-term inconveniences are long-term benefits, you won't become a casualty due to inaction.

What if one of the side effects of making the lifestyle changes found in this book is a long, healthy, active, independent, and robust family life? What if it's a life where you can be with your family more, not fear illness or disease, and spend more time living life versus planning life? What if it's a life where you can go biking with your family in the beauty of Ponderosa State Park in McCall, Idaho, or walk without hesitation eighty-eight flights of stairs in the Crystal & Fantasy Caves of Bermuda well into your nineties?

LIVE YOUR PLANS!

Now is always the time to stop *planning* that wellness life and start *living* that wellness life. Your body requires deliberate action to facilitate restoration and healing.

Find the recipe; cook the recipe.

Buy the equipment; use the equipment.

Pay the membership; use the membership.

Get the supplement; take the supplement.

Read the book; live the book.

Your body interprets plans without action as neglect—and neglect is a springboard for illness and disease. Just as a vacant house is subject to decay and rot, so too is an inert body at risk for illness and disease.

So I did it! I used what I knew and learned what I didn't know to bring healing, restoration, and realignment to my body. You can do the same.

But you have to *focus*—not on what you think you're losing but on what you'll be *gaining*. And trust me, there's a lot to gain. If you want to make a change that sticks, focus on your *wellness why*. If you're not sure what that is, that's a sign that you need to stop and think about it right now.

Your *wellness why* will keep you motivated when you find yourself headed to the drive-thru instead of going home after work to prepare a healthy meal. It will keep you going when your kids leave their bag of Halloween candy on the kitchen counter and you find yourself craving sweets after they've gone to bed. It will keep you going when you were supposed to meet your friend for a walk but she cancels at the last minute.

Your *wellness why* will help you stay strong when your friends start to pull away because they don't quite understand your new "healthy lifestyle."

It's not about doing it for them; it's about doing it for *you*. It's not enough to know you want to do it. For this to stick, you have to start with *why*.

HEALTH INTUITION AND SELF ADVOCACY

Curating a lifestyle around wellness versus trying to fit wellness into your lifestyle is the catalyst to long-term healing.

"Everything in moderation, including moderation" is a quote echoed by many. But what people fail to realize is that not everyone knows how to moderate.

Symptoms of autoimmunity, along with unwanted weight gain, hair loss, joint pain, eczema, acne, polycystic ovaries, exercise-induced asthma, seasonal allergies, uncontrolled blood sugar, decreased immunity, and gastrointestinal distress, are just some of the things I saw disappear completely or greatly reduced for me and for others when living in alignment with the principles in this book.

This is the reason that self-advocacy is so important. No one can advocate for you like you can. I first discovered the superpower of self-advocacy at the tender age of six. One evening, I challenged my mom about the need to complete my dinner. The culprit was the local fish that was on the plate. Telling her that it tasted bad, I pushed the plate away and refused to finish my dinner that night.

Just a few hours later, my pregnant mom, my dad, and my sister were crowding into the bathroom with bad cases of fish poisoning, as the islanders called it. Mom was rushed to the hospital. Because I didn't eat the fish, I was the only one who didn't get sick.

Decades later during my first pregnancy, my health intuition again helped me get through another potential health crisis. At 23 weeks gestation, I felt like something wasn't quite right with the pregnancy, and I asked my obstetrician to check my cervix during a routine visit.

Something was wrong, but I couldn't tell exactly what it was.

Her hand was already holding the door knob of the exam room, ready to move on to the next patient. I stood my ground, pleading for a physical exam, insisting that something just wasn't right. Eventually she returned to my side and discovered that my cervix had shortened dramatically in just a few weeks. Immediately I was placed on emergency hospital bed rest in an attempt to maintain the pregnancy.

Advocating for my health was not new. It was innate. Even when I returned to the hospital after my water broke a mere two weeks after being released from bed rest, I tirelessly advocated for admission to the labor and delivery unit just shy of 34 weeks. I intuitively knew that the well-being of my daughter and me were at stake.

A few months after all this began, after losing a frightful amount of blood and undergoing a life-threatening delivery, I delivered my prize of a four-pound, healthy baby girl.

It wasn't easy though. Notably, I had to engage in a verbal tug-of-war with my obstetrician. During the six weeks of hospital bed rest, I had to advocate for myself several times, including when a duplicate dose of a medicine was brought to my room for me to take. It also included negotiating with the nurses about the ideal time to administer my glucose tolerance test and when my groom turned the hospital linen closet into a makeshift nourishment pantry filled with fresh fruit, canned soup, granola bars, and snacks for the rest of the hospital stay.

I was convinced that the hospital menu was not designed to bring joy to my palate. I'm not even sure it was designed to bring proper nourishment to me or my unborn child's growing body.

One of the nurses advised me and gave me the permission I needed in order to survive bed rest. Soon after I checked in, she said, "Make the room your own." It was a lesson in wellness advocacy that I didn't know I needed.

So with trinkets from home and gifts from family and friends, my groom helped me decorate the room with flowers, pictures, cards, and some of my favorite things. There in the hospital room while my body was building a gift of a baby, my commitment to my own wellness advocacy was reborn.

I continued to advocate for me and my children's health, just like I had done in the hospital. That included disagreeing, annoying, and eventually enlightening health providers with my steadfast persistence and unwavering stance. I didn't necessarily want to challenge them, but I wanted to be worthy of being part of the conversation and having an opinion that always deserved to be heard.

I realized that our intuition is more important than we assume. We are all born with health intuition. Our intuition, I believe, is sharpened with continued use.

Sharpen your wellness intuition like a sword, and wave it around to work in your favor.

Whatever you do, don't take that intuition for granted.

We take care of our spouses, our children, and our parents. Then somewhere at the bottom, we see if we have enough time in the day to take care of ourselves.

Oh, and at the end of my journal entry, in the wee hours of that Bloody Valentine morning, I finished up by writing this: "If you were trying to send me a message, God, surely you didn't have to take me out to get me to listen. But now, I'm listening loud and clear."

The results of that intuitive listening are in the following pages of this book.

DR. LISA'S NOTES

» If you truly want change in any aspect of your life, you have to start with *why you want it.*
» Self-advocacy is your responsibility, and it cannot be outsourced.
» When it comes to your care, you are worthy of having an opinion, of having questions, of asking about alternatives.

WELLNESS PRESCRIPTION

» Identify your *wellness why.*
» What do you hope to gain? What do you hope to lose? Write it down, and read it every day.

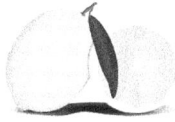

Chapter 4

FROM HEALTHCARE TO SELF-CARE: TIPS TO SHARPEN YOUR HEALTH ADVOCACY

Just because your insurance covers it doesn't mean it covers you.

If you're not going to advocate for your wellness and well-being, who's going to do it for you? Be an active patient. Ask questions during your doctors' visits. If you believe that something doesn't make sense or doesn't add up, then trust that inner knowing. Don't allow a nurse, nurse practitioner, doctor, or anyone else to take your vitals such as blood pressure without asking for the results. It's your blood pressure!

If you know your elevated blood pressure is more of an indication of the two-hour wait rather than chronic hypertension, then say something. Don't carry the energy or that frustration with you. Your care provider needs to know they're not respecting your time and that there are other factors to take into consideration.

The only way you can speak confidently about discrepancies in your blood pressure, for example, is if you know what your resting blood pressure is. That would come from checking your blood pressure at home on different days of the week and at different times of the day.

Sign up online to have access to your medical records. Keep a food journal or diary. A simple notebook with dates, foods consumed, and a separate section for how you feel after eating is a good start. If you feel off or that something is wrong, trust your instincts.

Buy a blood pressure monitor, blood glucose monitor, digital scale, and digital thermometer, and keep them in your home. If you don't know your numbers, it's going to be hard to advocate for yourself. You have to "know to glow." Wellness checks don't happen once a year; they happen every day.

If you're concerned about vitamin D deficiency or your immunity, or if you want to be more health empowered (hint: that should be everybody), have your vitamin D levels checked at least once a year. To be your own best advocate, you have to know.

If you're met with resistance or a physician who tells you that you must have a bone disorder to have access to that test, it may be time to get another doctor. This posture is a sign of sick care and has no place in health and wellness. There are also at-home vitamin D testing kits available that can be used in the comfort and privacy of your home.

Talk to trusted friends to get practitioner recommendations, and swap medical experiences and stories. Use your discernment when making decisions. Online forums may also be a good way to listen to others and share experiences.

Please note: While these groups should *not* be a source of medical advice, they can act as a source of baseline information and validation, and a place of support.

Create a medical board of directors. Your board should include the following:

- President (you)
- Gynecologist (if you own a vagina)
- Naturopath or integrative practitioner

If you want extra credit, add the following:

- Chiropractor
- Acupuncturist
- Holistic dentist

Remember, you may not be paying for your health visits and prescriptions out of pocket, but that doesn't mean they're free. Often there are unnecessary medications and procedures that lead to unnecessary complications you could have avoided.

Don't be scared to ask hard questions like the following:

"Why are you recommending this?"

"Is there a less invasive procedure that is just as effective?"

"Do you know of any non-drug alternatives?" (Don't stop here because unless you're dealing with an alternative practitioner, your doctor may not know.)

"Well, your insurance pays for it" is not a valid answer. That should come after your personal risk-benefit analysis. The fact that a provider has to pay for their new fancy machine has nothing to do with you.

True story: When I was pregnant with my second child, the doctor told me I had to have a surgical procedure in order to sustain a full-term pregnancy. No other options were mentioned in light of my previous medical history. I found out that my insurance company would pay for it.

Fortunately, I heard from a friend about a less-invasive, non-surgical procedure and mentioned it to my provider.

"What about this?" I asked. "Would that work just as well in my situation?"

To my surprise, her answer was yes. My provider told me that both procedures were equally effective, but she had never mentioned the other option.

The purpose of a medical insurance company has nothing to do with keeping you in the best health and shape of your life. *If people didn't get sick, hospitals, surgical centers, and the healthcare industry as a whole would not be booming moneymakers. A healthy patient is not a significant source of revenue.*

Of course, emergency medicine is sometimes needed. But sick care would be greatly reduced. That doesn't make the people behind the over-prescribed medicines and heavy-handed procedures bad people. It just means you need to know what those blind spots are and work harder to know what your role is in advocating for yourself accordingly.

Explore your options, and then make appropriate decisions. Just because your physician didn't tell you about it doesn't mean it doesn't exist. Conversely, just because your physician told you about it doesn't mean you should do it.

Under no circumstances should you allow yourself to be a victim of medical bullying. If your provider cuts you off mid-sentence and never has time for your questions, it may be time to get another provider.

If your provider refuses to listen to your concerns or has a patriarchal or matriarchal approach, it may be time to get another provider.

If your provider has the attitude of "only listen to me and do as I say," it may be time to get another provider.

Get a second opinion, but don't stop there. Three or more opinions may be warranted if you feel you're not getting the objective information you seek. By the way, even though validation from others feels good, it's not necessary to move forward in health and healing.

For example, if you've noticed that every time you have dairy you develop a case of acne, skin eruptions, and other ailments, then a negative allergy test result to milk is not a "green light" to plan an ice cream social for your upcoming birthday party.

Instead, recognize that all bodies are uniquely made, and celebrate that your body is built with a sophisticated alarm system decoded primarily by the first line of defense . . . *you*. Allergy tests are diagnostic tools that, although valuable, are not the end of the road.

Sensitivities, intolerances, and aversions are a thing. Learn to trust your body. The best gastroenterologists, internists, oncologists, or state-of-the-art machines can't teach you to trust your body. You have to do that.

That's how you go from healthcare (about them) to self-care (about you).

DR. LISA'S NOTES

» Healthcare is not self-care.
» Wellness checks should happen every day, not just once a year.
» What many people call "alternative medicine" used to be called "medicine." Holistic medicine is a more appropriate term.

WELLNESS PRESCRIPTION

» Assemble a medical board of directors. Be mindful to include practitioners and other experts of diverse holistic backgrounds and education.

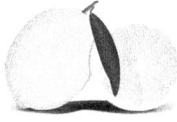

Chapter 5

FOOD, THE GUT, AND MINDFUL EATING

You can't call it "dietary restrictions" if it liberates you from illness and disease.

Do you know that your gut is also referred to as your second brain? That's because what happens in the gut not only affects your health but directly affects your thoughts, emotions, and actions. Likewise, what happens in the brain impacts what happens in the rest of the body. The gut-brain axis is like a busy highway that connects the cognitive and emotional centers of the brain with the intestines. So you see, you can't talk about true health without talking about the gut. And you can't talk about gut health without talking about the food that goes into it and all that comes with it.

Let's dive in.

If you were the embodiment of your dream car, what type of car would you be?

No matter what vehicle that is, I'm pretty sure the words *lemon* or *whoopty* wouldn't cross your mind. As such, when it comes to fueling or reenergizing your ride, it should be done with careful thought and consideration. Sure, you may think about buying discount gas from the new gas station down the street, but can you really trust that it won't drag down your car's performance?

Instead, you would probably go to a reliable gas station and get quality gas, even if it was out of your way. You may even be willing to pay a little more per gallon to get the right fuel.

You wouldn't connect a Corvette to a charging station, put regular gas in an Aston Martin, or fill up a Jaguar with diesel fuel.

Why not?

Well, because putting the wrong type of fuel in your car would be devastating.

That's exactly what happened when my groom inadvertently filled up our sedan with a full tank of diesel fuel. The car came to an abrupt stop, and we had to take notice. We made it about half a mile down the road before the car stopped on a small bridge on a particularly hot summer day.

Let me tell you, having any kind of car trouble is never fun. But stopping on a two-way bridge in the middle of summer with a small child takes things to a whole other level.

What's your bridge in life? You don't want to stop midway because you're filling up with the wrong fuel!

Your food is your fuel.

All food falls into one of two categories. Food is either (1) health-promoting or (2) disease-fostering.

Sure, you can walk the line and say that some foods are neither here nor there, but I think you get the point. It's up to you to know which category your foods fall into and what to do about it.

Wafting scents, well-crafted blog posts, holiday festivities, social calendars, spur-of-the-moment cravings, advertisements, and persuasions all have an impact on *what* you eat, *how* you eat, *when* you eat, and *how much* you eat.

To decide to govern yourself outside of our culture's societal norms can be a shock and a slap in the face to friends and family. In many cases, those changes are only accepted when you prove your own health to be vehemently and outwardly at risk. In this case, it doesn't seem like "an ounce of prevention is worth a pound of cure" rings true. It's more like "wait until it's severely broken, and then try to fix it."

Mindful eating means being present and paying attention to nutritional, medicinal, and physiological needs.

When people privately try to do the right thing, they often face the wrath of naysayers, bystanders, onlookers, and food pushers. These are the people who will barrage you at birthday parties, corner you at the church picnic, and try to make your vacation unpleasant until you cave and dive face first into a comfy plate of chocolate-glazed donuts.

In other words, while *reactive* healthcare is supported, employing *proactive* care is often insulted and ridiculed. Decide to skip dessert and you risk ruining events, hurting feelings, and perhaps risking friendships. Family and friends are often more accepting if there is an overt diagnosis, a few prescriptions, a chronic disease, or a near-death medical event to justify a change of diet.

There is a fundraiser for almost every type of disease you can think of, and people appropriately champion those causes. But if participants try to circumvent illness by making deliberate choices about what they eat and don't eat, they face snarky comments when they pass on the fudge and reach for the fruit.

We have accepted the notion that we are not the ones who govern our bodies but that someone else is in charge and more equipped—usually someone wearing a crisp, pressed white coat and carrying a stethoscope.

Many people wrestle for years with stomach issues, recurring indigestion, skin ailments, loose bowels, fibroids, arthritis, grogginess, stubborn weight loss, forgetfulness, restlessness, headaches, and more before the symptoms turn into something less innocent—something more sinister, something they can no longer ignore. Those early symptoms are the warning signs of decades of ongoing damage. Your body is so intelligent that it literally starts begging and pleading with you to make a change.

But instead, you pop an Alka Seltzer, reach for a Lactaid pill, or grab your regular bottle of pain reliever and cave in to the peer pressure when your bestie says you're "no fun" for skipping a big hunk of cheesecake.

It's this same mindset that encouraged a classmate of mine to feel comfortable enough to approach me at the gym and ask why I was still training. He blurted, "The university pageant is over, so why are you still working out?"

So instead of passing up the cheesecake, you pull up your chair and let your fork glide down a creamy slice, only interrupted by the occasional chocolate cookie crumble.

A food intolerance is not an allergy. But if you had an allergy, your bestie would meet it with understanding, acceptance, and even empathy.

Think about it—unless a medical professional diagnoses us with a food allergy, many of us continue to put ourselves through the horrid torment of skin rashes, recurrent vaginal candida, irritable bowels, skin rashes, achy joints, memory lapses, low energy, and more.

Here's a real concern: Oftentimes these milder symptoms foreshadow bigger problems down the line, including Crohn's disease, insomnia, cancer, arthritis, reproductive challenges, sleep disturbances, irritable bowel syndrome (IBS), diabetes, irritable bowel disease (IBD), coronary heart disease, and Alzheimer's.

When did we become a group of people who ignore our bodies' many cries for proper care in favor of societal acceptance or corresponding laboratory values?

If you learn to listen well to your body, you will be years and possibly even decades ahead of an avoidable medical emergency—the kind that leaves everyone in shambles and shaking their heads in disbelief, and makes them whisper, "She was so healthy. What do you think happened?"

Your body is screaming, shouting, and hoping that you avoid the pitfalls of dietary and lifestyle demise. But too often we ignore the screaming, much like when I pushed off the signs and symptoms of immune dysfunction, micronutrient depletion, and exhaustion, most likely skirting an autoimmune diagnosis while living a lifestyle I was too busy to change.

In my defense, I didn't think anything was wrong. I just thought I was balancing a full plate of entrepreneurship, parenting young kids, homeschooling, and travel, probably like you are balancing a variety of things right now.

Sure, maybe your plate is filled with different things, but my guess is that your plate is full nevertheless.

Yet still, I should have taken notice when I lost consciousness in a small airplane lavatory 35,000 feet above ground headed to Côte d'Azur, France. It should have been an uneventful trip to the bathroom. In a moment of what can only be described as superwoman reflexes, I unlatched the small door just before losing consciousness, eventually collapsing and slamming my shoulder against something hard that left a pretty bad wound. I woke up when the next passenger tried to open the lavatory door. My long, sprawling legs were pressed tightly against the door, preventing her from opening it all the way.

Take notice. Your body is speaking loudly. Are you too busy to listen?

It's an internal conversation that happens between you and your body. It won't be audible to friends, your spouse, or even Auntie Amy when you pass up her famous macaroni pie on Thanksgiving.

It's your body. You know the warning signs and what you're fighting for. Now it's time to choose mindfully and fight for it.

DR. LISA'S NOTES

» The gut is also known as the second brain.
» Food affects your health, thoughts, vitality, longevity, and emotions.

WELLNESS PRESCRIPTION

» What are some physical warning signs you need to address?

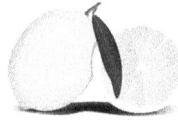

Chapter 6

NOURISH TO FLOURISH

*The problem with moderation is that most
people don't know how to moderate.*

"I'd rather die than change."

That's what he said as he sat across from me at the dinner table. And he was a smart guy too.

We were at a birthday party. I'm not even sure how the topic of diet came up, but that's what he said, and at that moment, I knew where he stood. The fact that he was a husband and a dad to three young kids didn't matter either.

Why are food habits some of the most difficult to break? A lot of "medical family history" is what we eat, learned to eat, saw our parents eat, and taught our kids to eat. Then there are the inherited bad lifestyle habits that go along with it. Those bad habits and lifestyle traits are passed down directly and indirectly like rotting seeds on a beloved family tree. Those seeds create plants that continue to propagate until someone is courageous enough to cultivate new seeds and change the quality of the fruit.

Why would someone rather die than change the way they eat? One of the first things we learn as babies is how to nourish. It happens at a subconscious level. From the time a baby is in utero, mom's amniotic fluid is flavored with different tastes from her diet, and a developing fetus can taste it.

The whole idea that "my child does not like___" should be switched to "my child has not learned to appreciate___," and then go from there. Most children are not born with an endearment for cruciferous vegetables, for example. Parents have to go through a cycle to introduce, reintroduce, and model over and over before the child actually gets it.

By the time that child becomes an adult and is told certain foods are inherently bad for health or they need to make a change, we're talking about many decades of unhealthy food conditioning. What's the point? It took you a while to get to this place, and it's going to take a while to find your way out.

To help you find your way, start with these important questions.

WHO

Who are you?

I don't mean things like I'm a forty-two-year-old single black female, a non-smoker who likes long walks on the beach and good foot rubs.

I mean what's your heritage? What's your family's medical history? Do you have any food allergies? Does eating beans give you noxious gas?

Who are you eating for?

This question should be easy to answer. You're obviously eating for yourself.

If you're growing a little human or humans inside you, you'll be eating for more than just yourself. During pregnancy, the calories you get are even more important because they are helping build one of the greatest miracles of life. If that's you, congratulations! Remember that eating for two only boils down to eating an extra 300 calories per day. Don't believe the hype!

WHAT

What Do I Eat?

Do you want to know what to eat? I thought you'd never ask. But first, remember this is not about deprivation; it's about liberation from unwanted pain, disease, illness, and suffering. Yes, to get there you have to pivot and remove some things from your plate. But you'll also get to add lots of nutrient-dense foods to the mix, some of which you may not have even known existed. What you'll gain in return is so much more. Before you delve in, take note that you have the power. And with that power, it's not about "what you *can't* have" but about "what you *choose* not to have."

If you're having difficulty trying to figure out what to cook, the good news is that there are lots of options, and I'm the right person to hold your hand and take you there.

You see, even though I started cooking in my single digits, I haven't always made the right decisions. I recall standing in the kitchen with my best friend after grade school one day, trying to figure out the recipe for Snickers candy bars.

Another time, when I was around ten, we fried sticky dough and carelessly dusted it with loads of cinnamon sugar.

My mom loves telling everyone the story of when she rushed home to make dinner after a long day at work to find that I had already made a huge gourmet salad complete with leftover meat, vegetables, and boiled eggs. I was around twelve at the time.

Fortunately, I eventually pivoted to making consistent healthier meals.

Years ago when I hosted in-person wellness cooking parties, I prepared three original healthy recipes for audiences of a dozen or more people at a time. During the event, I brought attendees into the kitchen to cook with me. My purpose was always to make healthy cooking tasty, approachable, and fun. I've used that same approach on numerous television shows, my own web series, live online events, and even while hosting my own event at my local Whole Foods.

Even so, I understand that when you're at home, bogged down with the responsibilities of life while trying to keep your kids from catching a bug from a child at school, cooking doesn't always feel like a cooking party. Mostly it can feel like another dreaded thing on the list of things you just don't want to do.

Even if you are initially motivated to "do the right thing," you can easily fall prey to the trap of getting entangled with foods that drag you down, weigh on your immunity, and make it hard to lose the "baby weight" even though your child is now sixteen and about to get her driver's license.

Whatever the reasons are, the options for those who don't want to cook or need some extra help getting healthy meals on the table are numerous. There are meal kits, food prep services, and more.

At the end of the day, are you filling your plate with whole, organic, life-giving foods versus ones that are life-robbing? Is your food free of artificial colors, sugars, and preservatives? Does your food mitigate disease or promote it?

Are you shopping grass-fed, pasture-raised, free range, and wild when possible? Is every meal accompanied by fresh vegetables and fruits? Can you pronounce all the ingredients in your food? Would your great-grand-mother recognize what you're eating as food? After eating, do you feel energized and upbeat versus down and withdrawn?

Reading food labels are an important aspect of nourishing to flourish. I'm sure you've heard the saying, "It's not what's on the outside; it's the inside that counts." Well, when it comes to getting the right type of food, if it comes in a bag, can, package, or whatever, it's not what's on the front label but what's on the back that really counts. To understand this, you have to understand food labels and how to read them.

In the United States, labels showing food ingredients are governed by the Food and Drug Administration (FDA). According to the FDA, ingredients are listed in the order of decreasing prominence. What that means is that for any package or food label you read, the first ingredient on the food label is what is in the highest quantity in that food, usually by weight. The ingredient on the bottom of the list is the least quantity.

While packaged food is not preferred, when eating in alignment with Being FINE, the first five ingredients on any food package should not include any grains, hydrogenated fats, sugars, or dairy. And nowhere should you see references to artificial colors or artificial flavors.

What's Eating You

You're probably reading this and thinking, "What do you mean?"

Don't be too quick to brush off this question.

Stick with me here. I don't mean to gross you out, but over three million people in the United States are affected by parasites. Most of those parasites are pinworms that live in the human gastrointestinal system. When you're affected by parasites, sorry to break it to you, but you're not just eating for yourself.

Parasites love carbohydrate-rich and sugar-laden foods. And since those parasites can't make their own food, you're eating for more than you know. Some of the paths to entry for parasites are eating under-cooked meats, swimming in lakes, drinking unclean water, and getting an insect bite.

As a result, a statement such as "I just have a sweet tooth" could mean that "my parasites love sugar, and I'm feeding their insatiable appetite." Not to be outdone, yeasts are unicellular organisms whose presence can bring unpleasant and sometimes disastrous effects on health. Hence, an overgrowth of yeast or candida can also cause a voracious appetite for sugar. While some yeast is common in everyone, candida overgrowth is of particular issue and affects many people.

Unfortunately, added sugar is present in almost all processed food items.

Signs of yeast overgrowth include recurrent yeast infections, sugar cravings, thrush, skin infections (ringworm, toe fungus, athlete's foot), GI symptoms, and more.

Some of the things that cause candida overgrowth are diets high in sugar, use of birth control, excessive alcohol consumption, and antibiotic use.

If you think you have been affected by parasites or yeast, it's important to not only starve them out by depriving them of their preferred food source (sugar and refined carbs) but also seek treatment. If you're well read and sure of what you're doing, you may be able to do that at home. There are many parasite cleanses and kits out there. You can find the best ones in natural food stores or with guidance from a holistic professional with expertise in this area.

Some natural antiparasitic herbs and foods include wormwood, black walnut, clove oil, oregano oil, garlic, and pumpkin seeds.

WHEN

When to Buy

When it comes to "when to buy," there are two *whens* to consider: when to go grocery shopping and when to buy things like fruits and vegetables.

The best time to go grocery shopping is when your stomach is satiated and the grocery store is not packed with people. If you're hungry, you'll pick up more high-caloric, nutrient-poor foods that don't serve you.

To avoid the after-work, after-school crowds, go early in the morning instead of after 5:00 p.m. You can also go shopping late at night or an hour or two before closing. The problem with the latter option, however, is that fresh produce is often picked over by then, and the fresh seafood and meat departments may already be closed. The busiest times at the grocery store are weekends and after 5:00 p.m. when many people get off work.

If the grocery store is filled with too many people, you may pick up items in a hurry without reading nutrition labels. In addition, you may miss items on your shopping list that you came for. Of course, when you do your grocery shopping online, things like this are less likely to be an issue.

When to Eat

For the majority of human history, our ancestors ate just one or two meals a day. These days, we call that "intermittent fasting," while our ancestors just called it life. The "you have to eat three square meals" mentality has robbed many people of the benefits that built-in food breaks can bring, which include autophagy, immune priming, cell repair, illness recovery, and more.

Intermittent fasting, or time-restricted eating (TRE), is identified by taking deliberate food breaks of twelve to sixteen hours between meals. During that time, eating is compressed to an eight-to-twelve-hour window. This is not just about caloric restriction. You're not trying to restrict the number of calories you eat during the window. However, your appetite will naturally become smaller. You will, of course, eat less food, and your metabolism will improve.

You can learn how to eat based on your body's own natural internal cues versus the rituals based on societal norms.

According to food historians, for much of history, people didn't eat breakfast. And do you know that the term *breakfast* means break the overnight fast? Fasting is a big part of human culture. Historically, some of the reasons people have fasted—and still do—include religious rituals, cancer treatment and prevention, seeking spiritual guidance, weight loss, improved mental clarity, blood sugar control, and general wellness practices.

As a result, rather than using terms such as breakfast, lunch, and dinner, try the terms first meal, second meal, and so on. They offer more freedom and flexibility to be conscious during your time of nourishment.

WHY

Why You Buy

Why do you buy the things you buy at the grocery store? Is it out of habit? Are your purchase decisions driven by convenience or by the ads that bombard you throughout your favorite TV show?

Why You Eat

Interestingly, people don't always eat just because they are hungry. So *why* are you eating? Are you eating:

- because you're bored, lonely, or depressed?
- because you feel pressured or don't want to hurt someone's feelings?
- because you're unconsciously feeding unknown parasites?
- as a matter of avoidance?
- because you want to socialize or celebrate?
- because the food is there?
- because somebody pissed you off?

Here are better reasons to eat:

- Genuine hunger
- For growth
- For cleansing
- To get well
- For energy
- To boost your immunity
- To gain or lose weight
- For longevity
- For nourishment

When it comes to grocery shopping to get FINE, keep these reasons at the forefront. Taste and palatability are important, but the ultimate goal is to nourish in order to flourish. Keep that goal top of mind, and it'll be easier to stick to your goals.

WHERE

Where to Buy

When it comes to buying whole foods, there are many options to consider. For the sake of keeping this section focused, I'm going to skip over restaurants for now because even though there are some healthy options out there, you just don't have control of what goes into your food.

Farmers' markets and grocery stores are much better options when buying life-giving versus life-robbing food. When I refer to life-giving food, I am referring to organic food sourced locally whenever possible. I am referring to wild-sourced (important for blueberries and fish), pasture-raised (poultry, eggs), grass-fed and finished (beef), antibiotic-free (all meats), non-GMO (across the board), grain-free, definitely gluten-free, and minimal dairy foods. Butter and ghee contain minimum casein (protein found in cow's milk) and lactose (a sugar found in cow's milk) and are well-tolerated in people who avoid dairy.

If you live in the United States, use these resources to help source the best food you can.

American Grassfed Association (AGA)

This website allows you to search producers of certified grass-fed beef that is pasture-raised, 100 percent foraged, and antibiotic-free.

BiodynamicFood.org

This is a resource for biodynamic food brands and farms. This is a bit more than farming organic food since biodynamic food practices are committed to holistic, non-chemical, sustainable, and regenerative farming practices.

LocalHarvest.Org

Use this website to find farms, farmers' markets, and community sourced agriculture (CSA) in your area.

Cornucopia.org

This nonprofit website keeps consumers abreast of ratings on certified organic products such as eggs and beef, and issues that may be affecting the organic community.

Where to Eat

Not only have we been programmed to ignore our bodies' innate cues when it comes to eating, but schedules and convenience have become more important than setting aside quality time to eat. This is such a pervasive problem that not even mealtimes are sacred anymore. Meals at dinner tables and breakfast nooks have been replaced with meals in drive-thrus, in parking lots, crouched over computers, at traffic lights, and on the couch in front of the TV.

The problem with this is not so much where you eat but what happens when human consciousness and nourishment are not aligned. Mindful eating happens in the absence of distractions such as phones, TVs, screens, and other devices. The battle for mealtime consciousness started in the 1950s with the advent of TV dinners, and we've been fighting hard ever since. Distracted eating can lead to unnecessary overconsumption of calories and dissociation of taste and quality.

If possible, make time to eat meals each day away from the television, computers, electronics, work commitments, and other distractions. It may seem weird, but eating at breakfast tables, dining room tables, and even outdoors is favored and ideal if you want to get FINE.

Try this. In certain countries, lunchtime is known as siesta. It's literally time to eat lunch and then nap. In some of my previous travels to Europe, I encountered several instances where stores were closed during lunchtime.

In Paris and Buenos Aires, for example, I often saw people dining in nature's original dining room—a patch of grass—while enjoying the company of others during meals.

There can be challenges! If you have young kids at home, it's hard to drink a cup of tea while it's hot. It's even harder to sit down to eat dinner mindfully. Keep working on it though. At some point, I promise it will get better.

I'm sure you've heard of distracted driving, but have you heard of distracted eating? Distracted eating is eating while engaging in another activity. Distracted eating activities include driving, talking on the phone, scrolling on the internet, watching TV, and more.

This will take some practice, but when you're at home, reserve eating for places inside the kitchen and dining areas. Avoid working lunches while you're hunched over a computer. Even if you only have ten minutes, you can be present and fully dedicated to experiencing your food in those ten minutes.

The colors, textures, tastes, and smells are all important when you're having a mindful eating experience. Distracted eating, on the other hand, leads to overeating and unwanted weight gain.

DR. LISA'S NOTES

» Keep the five questions in mind as you grocery shop and eat meals.
» Learn how to eat based on your body's own natural internal cues versus rituals based on societal constructs.

WELLNESS PRESCRIPTION

» Every day, set aside time for distraction-free meals (away from phones, TV, etc.). There are bonus points if you eat at least one meal outside each day.

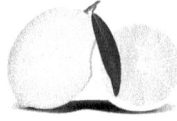

Chapter 7

THE GROCERY GAME

When I realized that the money I was saving on groceries was actually being spent on co-pays, I started to eat differently. Your livelihood matters, but your life matters more.

When thinking about grocery shopping, remember that you don't actually have to go into a grocery store to do it. The point is to source your food from reliable sources. Farmers' markets can be a great resource for fresh fruits, vegetables, and even pasture-raised and grass-fed meats. But be careful—"fresh" does not mean "organic." So talk to the vendors and farmers, and make sure their food values align with yours.

While farmers' markets provide a great opportunity to shop local and get some fresh air, just because it's sold at a farmers' market doesn't mean it's good for your body or good for you. Be leery of all the same types of wellness traps you can get at a traditional grocery store. That includes things such as artificial colors, artificial flavors, hydrogenated fats, GMOs, hidden sugars, and more. In particular, avoid non-organic produce, cakes, pastries, breads, jams, and jellies that have way more sugar than they have fruit.

GROW YOUR OWN

Besides shopping at farmers' markets, gardening is another way to have access at your fingertips to fresh produce and herbs. You don't even have to grow a lot. In addition, container gardening offers accessibility for those with limited space. You can start small and then go from there. Herbs and vegetables, including spinach, basil, lettuce, thyme, and bell peppers, make great plants for beginning gardeners.

Here are some other benefits of growing your own garden.

It's more affordable. Let's face it. Healthy eating doesn't have a reputation for being low cost. But the truth is that if you're not going to invest in healthy eating habits, you're going to pay for unnecessary prescriptions, surgeries, and a lifetime of inconvenience. It's your choice. The point is that growing your own food makes healthy eating and shopping more affordable.

It teaches kids responsibility. A family garden is a great way to get "all hands on deck" while teaching kids responsibility. Children as young as two can help with tasks such as weeding, watering plants, and selecting what crops to grow. It's a rewarding experience all around.

It burns calories. Gardening burns between 200 and 400 calories an hour, and no treadmill or weights are required.

It's a science lesson. Forget about learning about ecosystems in science books. Organic gardens have a plethora of organisms that interact all the time, and it's a marvel to watch and learn.

You can grow what you want. One of the most delightful things about having a family garden is growing exactly what you want and when you want it (climate permitting, of course). If you like carrots, grow some carrots. If you don't like arugula, skip it and grow spinach instead. It's your family garden, and you get to pick and choose what you want to grow. If you have young kids, get them involved, and find out what they want to grow. You may be surprised. Kids often want to eat what they grow!

You can share what you don't eat. One of the things that's great about gardening is sharing the harvest with neighbors and friends. It's quite a joy and always brings a smile to their faces.

You actually need less space than you think. If you're thinking about starting a family garden, don't let space be a hindrance. Container gardening and vertical space gardening are ideal options if you're short on space.

You make fewer trips to the store. Growing your own produce means you'll make fewer trips to the grocery store, which is always a good thing. If you're in need of some spring greens for the next salad, just go out and snip some. No car ride or gas money is required.

It fosters family bonding. Having a family garden is not just about the food; it's about family. Tilling, growing, toiling, and reaping together create memories that will last a lifetime.

It's just good for you. Having an organic family garden means more fruits and veggies to enjoy, which will help boost immunity. Gardening also leads to more sun exposure, exercise, time outdoors, family bonding, and lots of smiles. All these things can have a tremendous positive impact on your health.

THE DIFFERENCE BETWEEN NON-GMO AND ORGANIC FOOD

I know you're trying to make better decisions and eat healthier foods. But let's face it. If you don't know what you're looking for, shopping at grocery stores will be confusing.

First, I recommend sourcing your food from local and organic sources whenever possible. That includes shopping at farmers' markets, community-supported agriculture (CSA) markets, and natural grocers. It includes growing your own.

Organic items are naturally derived and not synthetic. Even so, it's important to note that buying organic doesn't necessarily mean the food is pesticide- or herbicide-free. It does mean that if any pesticides are used, they are natural. Also, the land used to grow those crops should be pesticide-free for the last three years. In addition, any equipment used to apply those organic pesticides should not have been used to apply synthetic pesticides for that same duration of time.

When items are labeled non-GMO certified, it means the seeds used to grow those items and any feed used have not been genetically modified.

Remember that non-GMO certification has nothing to do with the possible use of pesticides, chemicals, or fungicides in food. Glyphosate is a powerful herbicide found in weed killers such as Roundup, and it is a nemesis to health. Glyphosate has been linked to ailments such as cancer. It is also an endocrine disruptor known to affect the gut microbiome. Monsanto, the manufacturer of Roundup, was ordered to pay billions of dollars to gardeners, farmers, and groundskeepers due to damage to their health.

In the gut, glyphosate binds to metals that gut flora need to function optimally. When certain bacteria are limited in your gut, you can lose the ability to digest things such as gluten and dairy. That has been linked to the skyrocketing increase of celiac disease, dairy allergies, and food intolerances over the years.

Glyphosate is sprayed pre-harvest on crops such as wheat, barley, oats, and rye in a process known as desiccation. The herbicide is applied right before crops are picked in order to dry out the crops and speed up harvest time. Other crops commonly sprayed with glyphosate include but are not limited to almonds, apples, grapes, rice, lentils, and chickpeas. Going organic can lessen glyphosate exposure since organic crops are not treated or grown with glyphosate.

GMO crops can be organic. Organic crops can be GMO. At the same time, buying organic doesn't mean your food is pesticide-free as some pesticides are approved in organic farming. The best course of action is to do your best to make sure your food is both non-GMO and certified organic. Although that doesn't mean you're 100 percent in the clear, it does reduce your overall exposure and potential health risk, and that's a good thing.

To lower the risk of GMO foods, buy foods that are certified non-GMO. As a rule, less than 1 percent of genetic modification is allowed in foods labeled non-GMO.

For meats, you should focus on organic, pasture-raised chicken and poultry (raised using non-GMO feed), wild fish, and grass-fed, grass-finished lamb and beef. Eggs should be organic and pasture-raised. If pork is part of your diet, pasture-raised pork using non-GMO feed is preferred. Avoid conventionally raised meat as much as possible. For everything else, shop both non-GMO and organic.

The More You Know, the More You Glow!

Do you know that corn and soy are the most GMO foods?

HOW TO GROCERY SHOP

The invention of grocery stores was a wonderful thing. It meant we could shift our energy from being hunter gatherers to pursuing other passions and interests. It also meant that we saved energy and time looking for food. Most people would agree that the convenience of grocery stores is a wonderful thing. But did you know that how you grocery shop and what you shop for are also tied to wellness and well-being?

You may argue that there is nothing to learn when it comes to grocery shopping. You just set your budget, walk into the store, and "shop 'til you drop." However, when you're shopping to support a healthy lifestyle, it's not as simple as just walking into the grocery store and grabbing items off the shelf like you're on an episode of *Supermarket Sweep*.

While certain grocery brands have more bountiful organic and natural food selections, just shopping at a trusted grocery store is not enough for optimal wellness. You also have to put the right things in your cart if you want to win at the grocery store game. After all, last time I checked, organic white sugar is not a health food, even though you can find it at a health store.

Just because it's organic doesn't mean it's good for you.

WHAT TO BUY

Winning at the grocery game begins at home. Here's how.

Step 1. List the things you need. Whether you make an online grocery list, use a notes app, or just write a list on a piece of paper, the key is to start your grocery list before you even step foot into the store. Ideally, you would start making the shopping list at least a few days before you need to go grocery shopping. Once an everyday item is used up, a replacement should immediately be added to the list. That, of course, is the easy part.

Step 2: Add healthy staples. Things like cauliflower rice, raw nuts, carrot sticks, unsweetened almond butter, wild shrimp, pasture-raised chicken breasts, eggs, frozen vegetables, and wild canned fish adds flexibility and can really help.

Step 3: Plan your healthy menus. Next, decide what meals and snacks you'll be making over the next one to two weeks. Ideally, you will start with a wellness meal plan. Use this book, magazines, cookbooks, blogs, websites, and trusted websites to collect whole food, non-inflammatory recipes, and other inspiration on what to prepare.

A long-time blog reader and friend recently mentioned to me that a refresher about exactly which foods are inflammatory would be beneficial. Remember, this process is not about vilification but about education that can further benefit your health liberation. That's because each bite is either a catalyst to disease or a liberator from it.

So let's get to it.

Exposure to inflammatory foods can cause chemical reactions in your body due to your body trying to heal itself from damage. That is a result of the immune system being activated and doing what it's supposed to do. If inflammation in the body goes unchecked or is long-term, it can lead to illness and disease. As a matter of fact, the majority of diseases are caused by underlying inflammation.

In preparation for grocery shopping, use the list below to keep you on task. This list is not intended to be all-inclusive but rather a selection of foods and food groups that are notorious for causing inflammation and don't deserve to have a space in your cart.

While the connection to these foods and inflammation is well-documented, this list is not without debate. So consider your own dietary specifications, and use at your discretion.

Foods that cause (and can cause) inflammation:

- Refined sugar
- Grains (wheat, rye, barley, corn, rice, oatmeal, etc.)
- Conventionally raised meat
- Dairy
- Gluten
- Artificial dyes
- Artificial colors
- Refined oils

- GMO foods
- Conventional eggs
- Processed foods

I've also included some recipes at the end of this book as part of the Be FINE program.

FINE foods are grain-free, mainly dairy-free (with an exception for pasture-raised butter or ghee), organic, non-GMO, free of artificial colors and preservatives, and contain little refined sugar. We'll talk more about "why" in the inflammation chapter.

Grains are *not* in alignment with the Be FINE lifestyle. This means that corn, wheat, rye, rice, oats, spelt, and barley should not have a permanent home on your plate. It leaves lots of room for a plethora of organic fruits, colorful vegetables, and responsibly sourced protein.

The good news is that when it comes to starches, there are many other options such as quinoa, buckwheat, sweet potatoes and true wild rice, not to be confused with wild rice blends and mixes.

If you have issues with GI distress and are not vegetarian or vegan, avoid foods and recipes made with legumes for the first ninety days. That includes but is not limited to peanuts, peanut butter, beans (black, navy, red, white), chickpeas, garbanzo beans, lentils, coffee, and soy products. Green peas and green beans are more nutritionally aligned with vegetables and are not true legumes; hence, they are allowed.

The reason to exercise caution with legumes is because they contain a high amount of lectin and phytic acid, which are known anti-nutrients that can bind to ingested nutrients and tissues, and can cause irritation in the gut. Many people have a condition known as leaky gut, which leads to other ailments such as mood disorders, skin conditions, micronutrient deficiencies, autoimmune diseases, gut disorders, food allergies, and food sensitivities. While other foods contain lectin and phytic acid, legumes can be a big trigger.

If you're trying to truly heal the body, you have to heal the gut. Limiting possible irritants can aid in your understanding of how those foods may be affecting you and lead to some assemblage of healing.

Everybody handles lectins and hence legumes differently. But you don't know what you don't know. So my recommendation is to remove them, at least initially, and see how you do. After the first ninety days, slowly add legumes back in as tolerated, taking note of how your body responds to such changes.

Here's a tip: If beans are part of your diet, under no circumstances should you ever cook them in a slow cooker. All beans naturally contain a compound known as phytohaemagglutinin, a form of lectin. Slow cooking doesn't get temperatures high enough to break down this natural toxin. As a result, people can get severely ill, demonstrating symptoms such as vomiting, diarrhea, and abdominal cramping.

While I'm known for my tasty, mostly clean, non-inflammatory, and plant-heavy omnivorous recipes and videos, I went back and forth about whether or not I should include recipes in this book. And here is why. People often want to skip forward to the food without first understanding the foundational principles of *why* they should eat as described. That's the reason so many diets fail, which, for the record, I'm not a fan of.

While you'll be happy to know that I did include many delicious recipes, please don't skip forward to them just yet. In order to make a lasting change that will take you from surviving to thriving, it's imperative that you read this book all the way through in order to get results that stick.

Step 4: Shop the perimeter of the grocery store. When grocery shopping, if you start mindlessly headed down the aisles, you're grocery shopping the wrong way. Always go to the perimeter of the grocery store first. That is where they sell fresh fruits, vegetables, nuts, seeds, wild caught fish and seafood (including fatty fish), and pastured and grass-fed meats. You're not trying to go fat free here. Remember that the brain is 60 percent fat, so the body needs fat to function. The freezer section is also a good resource for quality protein and flash-frozen organic fruits and vegetables for longer storage and greater affordability.

Step 5: Read nutrition labels. Learning to read nutrition labels is super important when playing the grocery store game. Things to take note of are serving sizes, added colors, preservatives, sugars, and anything you can't pronounce. The serving size tells you how many nutrients, calories, and additives you can expect per serving.

For example, snacking on a pack of granola bars may seem like a healthy idea at first until you read the nutrition label and realize that a serving size is just one bar and you had planned on eating the entire pack of two as a snack. And those commercial "healthy" granola bars often contain a hefty dose of sugar or corn syrup.

A NOTE ABOUT SHOPPING WITH KIDS

Grocery shopping with children can make an arduous task even more involved. So if you can, go at it alone. As a homeschooling mom as of this writing, I know that this is often not possible. So I get it. Be that as it may, grocery shopping is a love-it-or-hate-it task for many. But whether you love it or hate it, planning is key when shopping with kids.

Here are five tips on how to grocery shop tear-free with kids.

1. First, Fill Their Tummies

If you're like most parents, you may have to take the kids to the grocery store with you. So you've got your shopping list and car keys, and you've set the house alarm, but did you give your kids something to eat? Always make sure the kids eat before you head out the door. The saying "never shop on an empty stomach" especially applies to kids. Taking your children to the grocery store while they're hungry is like taking them to Disneyland and refusing to buy any tickets. If you do that, something is likely to blow up. Be prepared for a grumpy, cranky, whiny, cute little person(s) to make things very difficult for you and loud entertainment for others. So . . . feed them first!

2. Establish Some Ground Rules

As with any other situation, you have to let your expectations be known. If you waltz into the grocery store and hope your kids will be well-behaved—well, that may just not happen. So establish some rules before you get to the store. Let your "little people" know what they can and can't do. Example: Are they allowed to make grocery selections and/or put things in the cart? Are they allowed to run around the grocery store chasing each other like cats and dogs? You know, this is all the normal stuff. If you establish these ground rules initially, you will keep the surprise factor to a minimum.

3. Assign Everyone a Task

Make sure to give your kids jobs to do when they go shopping with you, and then they won't feel so bored. Depending on the age of the kids, someone can be in charge of placing items in the cart, another for pushing the cart, someone to pay the clerk, and someone else to check items off the list. Of course, if you are shopping with babies, just ask the baby not to cry and to be cute. That is easier to achieve when the baby has been fed, is well-rested, and has a dry diaper.

4. Make It Fun

Grocery shopping with kids can really be a lot of fun. The grocery store is a great place to practice letter recognition and colors. Play games like "I spy" and matching. Ask questions such as "Are these items the same or different?" Help them practice their cognitive skills. Your child can practice counting by helping you get the desired number of items in the cart. Say, "I need five cans of green beans. Can you help mommy get five cans of green beans into the cart?" If your grocery store has a seafood section with live lobsters or crabs, go visit it. Make an event out of it.

5. Use Props, and Keep It Interesting

Modern grocery stores are full of fun things to keep kids entertained. There are digital scales, personal scanners, and sometimes even little shopping carts. The key is to show the child what to do and monitor them to make sure they are indeed helping and not deterring.

I did not say that the trip to the grocery store would be short, but it can be tears-free. And at the end of the day, having a tears-free mommy and tears-free children will make everyone happy!

FOR THOSE WHO HATE GROCERY SHOPPING

You're only as healthy as the meals you cook and what you eat. Over the years, I have written original recipes, done live cooking demos, and shared my holistic food ways on my own online web series and TV screens across the nation. People often tell me, "I don't have time to grocery shop" or "I hate grocery shopping."

Years ago, there were not many other options than to suck it up and do the grocery shopping yourself. These days, you can tap into grocery shopping apps, store delivery services, and more. A plus is that when you grocery shop online, you can intentionally skip unhealthy snack aisles and the checkout line that is often strategically surrounded with sugary and heavily salted snacks.

In addition, there are reliable mail order food companies that will allow you to source everything from fresh wild seafood; grass-fed, grass-finished beef; and even olive oil. You just have to know where to go—and as you know, *the more you know, the more you glow!*

TIPS FOR BUYING OLIVE OIL

Do you know that more than 70 percent of olive oil in American grocery stores is actually fake? Olive oil adulterating is a huge business. Many olive oils are often mixed with lower-quality oils such as soybean, vegetable, canola, sunflower, and more.

Do your due diligence, and make sure you are buying olive oil from a reliable source. Thoroughly research the company you're buying olive oil from. You can also buy directly from the producer to minimize your likelihood of getting fake oils.

Looking for the name "extra virgin" on the bottle versus just "olive oil" can be an indication of a higher-quality oil. Look on the label for the country or region of source. Good olive oil will be stored in a dark or opaque bottle so sunlight doesn't get through. That is important because light can affect the quality of olive oil by causing deterioration. So always keep your olive oil in a dark place.

FOOD FABLES

Now that you've picked up this book, you're opening yourself up to different thoughts about health and food rather than the ones you learned both consciously and unconsciously. When you were a child, your mom may have "branded" you as a picky eater or never liking vegetables. Your dad may have told friends and family that you were like him and didn't like spinach. Whether you're aware of it or not, you held on to that story. You got attention for that story. You may have even carried your food story with you into adulthood. What is your food story? You may have more than one. Take a few moments to make note of them here.

MY FOOD STORY...

_____

_____

_____

_____

Maybe you were always told that you had to "clean your plate." Maybe your food story is tied to fond memories of having glazed donuts every Sunday, and that made you feel loved. Or maybe, just maybe, you were unconsciously taught that going on diets is a normal state of being. Perhaps your momma told you that all women in your family carry the "weight of the plate" in their hips and thighs once they hit forty. Behavior personified shouldn't be misinterpreted for genetics.

Whatever your food beliefs are, you need to tackle them head on before you dive into the rest of this book.

List them. Write them down. Go straight to the source or risk of having "food fables" sabotage the dietary truths that can lead to wellness wins.

DR. LISA'S NOTES

» Grocery shopping is more than about picking up groceries and dropping them in your cart.
» Don't be provoked into making food choices that don't support your mission to Be FINE.
» The foods you buy can either build you up or break you down.

WELLNESS PRESCRIPTION

» Survey your kitchen, and remove anything that doesn't support your wellness mission. Your home is your haven. Superman would never stock kryptonite in his kitchen, so why would you?

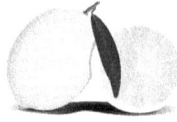

Chapter 8

FOOD–THE GOOD AND THE BAD

If it runs in your family, you can run past it.

Some people say there are no good or bad foods, and I agree—up to a point. While you may not categorize them as good or bad, there are pro-inflammatory foods and anti-inflammatory foods. There are disease-causing foods and health-promoting foods, energy-giving foods and energy-depleting foods, as well as age-promoting foods and anti-aging foods. There are foods that promote long life and longevity and, quite simply, other foods that don't.

We're eating things that our great-grandparents would not recognize as food, and then we're perplexed when the body opts to use those foods as building blocks for illness and disease.

You can beat around the bush if you want to and pretend that none of these things exist, but it will cost you.

It's romanticism to lament on how food used to be. The days when portion sizes were half what they are now, GMOs were nonexistent, and poultry didn't have to be labeled "free range" because it naturally was. Beef was obviously grass-fed, and wild-caught fish were just labeled "fish." Everything was non-GMO, free-range, grass-fed, and, of course, wild by nature's design.

Just stop and think about that for a second. What's being labeled organic, wild, non-GMO, locally grown food is not just how food *used* to be, it's how food is *supposed* to be. Farm-raised, genetically modified salmon, for example, didn't even exist as an industry until the 1980s. Today, as much as 75 percent of salmon sold worldwide is farm-raised. What's even crazier is that consumers have to pay more for how food used to be and still should be.

Speaking of food labels, always read them with both eyes open. That is because they're deceiving. For example, there are several additives and "bad for you" ingredients that are legally exempt from labeling requirements.

These exempt ingredients may be present in "low quantities." They include ingredients added for product enhancement such as added colors and flavor extracts.

What does all this mean?

It means that consumers can no longer be just consumers. You need to promote yourself to the level of an amateur food scientist if you want to "thrive, not just survive" in this modern-day world. Knowing how to properly read nutrition labels brings you one step closer to this.

But let's be honest—it's draining to talk about how life used to be in the "good ol' days." So I won't spend more time talking about that here. For the purposes of this book, your energy is best utilized not focusing on how things were but on how you need to be *right now*.

I'm not a fan of diets and dieting, but there's a reason why diets such as Keto, Mayr, Paleo, Whole 30, and Wheat Belly all include some level of wheat and/or grain modification. This is not by coincidence.

Some of these lifestyles/diets are rather new, but others, like the Mayr lifestyle, have existed for over a hundred years.

The truth is that the majority of people have a relentless addiction to starchy carbohydrates and inflammatory grains. As a matter of fact, if given the choice between a piece of bread or chicken, bread wins by far.

The problem is that foods such as rice, cookies, bread, pasta, and oats are notorious for their negative effect on insulin, glycemic response, and metabolism. Insulin spikes in particular are the foundation of many diseases and conditions.

Dr. William Davis discusses this in his popular book *Wheat Belly*, which notes the genetic changes that wheat has gone through over the centuries. And if you haven't guessed yet, these changes have had a devastating effect on our collective health. Genetic modification has been linked to increased intestinal permeability, autoimmune conditions, inflammatory diseases, cancer, and more.

This makes sense when you look at the growing number of people suffering from allergies, food sensitivities, skin disorders, asthma, autoimmune diseases, and other conditions at a devastatingly rapid pace. Much of the unnecessary suffering has nothing to do with family history. They are environmental and lifestyle-led maladies.

"Everything in moderation" is a quote that is often thrown around like ketchup packets at a fast-food restaurant. The problem with "everything in moderation" is that people don't know how to moderate.

Most people have a food moderator button that is broken, leading them down a path to certain destruction. If your moderator button is broken, who's going to tell you?

For those with a broken moderator button, there is no moderation. Just like some people are addicted to illicit drugs, alcohol, and unhealthy behaviors, others are just as similarly addicted to foods such as sugar, pasta, cake, and bread. It would be absurd to ask someone who identifies as an alcoholic to limit themselves to just one glass of wine. Similarly, no such limits are of value in the case of a food addiction.

These are highly volatile foods that may seem harmless on the surface, but for many they can be just as addictive as any street drug. The difference is that you don't need a dealer, and you don't have to hang out on shady corners to get your next hit. Nope, the stuff is all around you at grocery checkout lines, airports, conveniently located vending machines, and gas stations. These trigger foods ignite fires and wake up sleeping genes, and then "family history" gets to take all the credit for causing generational illness.

The truth is that genes can be turned on and off (this is called "gene expression"). Think of genes as the wiring in a house that controls all the lights and appliances. How you live, what you eat, and what you surround yourself with can either turn those genes on or off. Your genes are not the problem. Just because you're "wired" doesn't mean those genes have to "fire." It's really up to you.

WHAT'S THE DEAL WITH GLUTEN?

When most people think about gluten, they're referring to the gluten found in wheat. However, it's not just wheat that contains gluten; other grains that contain gluten include barley, rye, triticale, farro, spelt, and kamut. The gluten found in these grains is what causes concern for those with celiac disease and gluten sensitivities. Other grains such as rice and corn may be considered "gluten-free" because they contain a different kind of gluten that is tolerated and considered harmless by many. But, just because you're not aware of harm, doesn't mean that it's not there.

Wheat gluten contains two proteins—gliadin and glutenin—that are attached by amino acids. When wheat gluten is combined with water, these bonds impart a sticky yet chewy texture to breads, cereals, and baked goods that makes them so delicious.

It's the job of the digestive system to break this bond and make gluten digestible. The problem is that many people are unable to break those chemical bonds, and the chains of amino acids move unbroken into the small intestine, causing problems in the gut.

At the time of writing this book, one in every 133 Americans has been diagnosed with celiac disease, an autoimmune disorder that treats the gluten found in wheat as a foreign invader. Scientists estimate a larger number of people have undiagnosed celiac, and even more people are gluten intolerant or have non-celiac gluten sensitivity. The latter is even more frustrating since clinicians easily miss it, and available testing is often unreliable.

There are several clinically documented studies of *gliadin* (the protein found in gluten) crossing the gastrointestinal wall and blood-brain barrier. That may cause inflammation and disease even in non-celiac patients and people with no noted gluten sensitivity.

Having no visible outward symptoms of gluten sensitivity does not mean you're in the clear. Humans are highly adaptive. Bodies become accustomed to years of food abuse. Symptoms may present only at a microscopic level for years before an explosive big reveal when the body reaches its limit.

It's the gift and curse of adaptation that makes humans so magnificently made. Not realizing that outward manifestation is not necessary for the presence of illness or disease, people will often say, "But I've eaten this food for years and never had a problem." It's similar to how a lack of awareness of gravity doesn't mean it does not exist. The body is like an orchestra, and other musicians will often step up and overcompensate so the show can go on.

You probably know someone who went to see their doctor for a routine visit and returned with more than they had bargained for. But because they initially did not exhibit any outward symptoms of disease, everything came as a surprise.

Besides the issue of gluten, cross reactivities also occur with certain foods. Foods such as dairy are structurally similar to gluten, and antibodies will often elicit the same or similar reactions as if you were eating gluten itself.

Research shows that at least half the people who are sensitive to gluten also have cross-sensitivities to other foods. The damage caused to the gut by eating gluten and processed grains can lead to dairy sensitivity as well. Below is a list of foods that are cross-reactive with gluten:

- Dairy
- Corn
- Rice
- Oats
- Coffee
- Millet
- Yeast

The problem is that people who avoid gluten or decide to eat "gluten-free" look for comfort in gluten-free communities and groups littered with dubious gluten-free resources, recipes, and information. These foods can be filled with dairy, GMO-treated grains, and gluten-free food alternatives that offer comfort and familiarity but may be no better than the offending foods themselves. At the same token, food manufacturers add artificial flavors, thickening agents, artificial colors, and highly processed sugars to produce familiar textures and taste.

For example, corn is the most commonly grown crop in the United States, and the majority of it is genetically modified. Rice, another grain, has growing concerns over arsenic contamination. Oats, while naturally gluten-free, are often contaminated with wheat, and unless properly labeled cannot be considered gluten-free. These options can increase postprandial (after a meal) glycemic response, which has been linked to type 2 diabetes and obesity.

These gluten-free foods may offer some initial relief, but as time goes on, you find yourself right back where you started. The weight starts to creep back in, bloating ensues, and headaches and skin issues rebound until you find yourself with a growing list of ailments and complaints that the "gluten-free diet" just didn't work.

The best gluten-free foods are not labeled "gluten-free." The most nutritious foods are fresh, organic fruits and vegetables, nuts, seeds, and responsibly sourced and raised (wild, pasture-raised, grass-fed) fish, meats, and protein.

If you're considering removing gluten from your diet, it may seem counterintuitive, but avoid the so-called "gluten-free aisle." For the most part, those foods are stuffed with empty calories, packed with filler grains, and usually devoid of much beneficial nutrition.

Here's a quick story for you. A few years ago, as I stood in a buffet line with an acquaintance, I noticed that she served herself traditional lasagna. At the next station, she selected various gluten-free baked breads. At the next stop, she scooped out another piece of traditional pasta casserole. Curious, and thinking she may have inadvertently selected gluten-filled food by mistake, I mentioned that some items on her plate were not gluten-free. I did that in case she was indeed trying to embark on a new lifestyle.

She told me that she was aware and was opting for the gluten-free items to "balance out her plate" since those items were "healthier." Here's the truth: Carb-loaded, grain-filled breads are not healthy, whether or not they contain gluten.

You might as well just eat a big bowl of sugar. Okay, just kidding! Don't do that.

WHAT DO I EAT?

In truth, for much of human civilization, many unhealthy items were not part of anyone's diet. So just think of it as going back to how things used to be.

Keep in mind that you'll also get to add lots of nutrient-dense foods in return, foods you may not even know existed.

As an added benefit, you'll be able to win big with less effort in the battle of the bulge. Begin to make the necessary changes now, and in return you'll get so much more. Before you delve in, take note that you have the power. And that power is not about what you can't have; it's about *what you choose to eat.*

If you're having difficulty trying to figure out what to cook, the good news is that there are lots of options, and I'm the right person to show them to you. I realize that as much as cooking is my thing, it may not be yours. Or maybe you like to cook but tend to cook a lot of the wrong things.

When you're at home, bogged down with the responsibilities of life, cooking doesn't always feel fun. It can feel like another dreaded task on the list of things you just don't want to do.

Even if you're initially motivated to do the right thing, you can easily fall prey and get in an entanglement with foods that drag you down. You'll compromise your immunity and make it hard to lose those extra pounds you've been trying to shed.

Services, including home-delivered meal kits, are a valid option. They provide all the ingredients you need to easily and conveniently make healthy meals at home. Just be sure to pay attention to ingredients and portion sizes. Whether you're shopping at the grocery store or buying meal kits and ready-to-eat dinners online, you must be mindful of what you're putting into your body.

Non-Grain Alternatives to Bread, Pasta, and Rice

Bread

Cooked sweet potato rounds
Lettuce and large leafy greens
Nut-based breads and wraps
Eggplant slices
Nori
Paleo-labeled breads
Cassava-based/tapioca-based breads

Pasta

Soba noodles (if tolerated)
Shirataki noodles
Spiralized noodles using zucchini, sweet potato, and more
*Legume-based pastas (i.e., lentils)

Note: For those with underlying gastrointestinal (GI) disorders and distress, I recommend removing legumes for the first ninety days. Take note of how your body responds to a legume-free lifestyle, and adjust accordingly. If you decide to include legume pastas as part of your plan, look out for added binders, grains, fillers, and additives in these pasta alternatives. Lentils are at a high risk of cross contamination with crops containing gluten.

Rice

Wild rice (not wild rice mix) – true wild rice is not rice but rather the seed of a grass

Riced vegetables (cauliflower, broccoli)

Quinoa (naturally high in protein, quinoa is a seed, not a grain)

Non-Grain Starches

Potatoes of various colors and varieties (purple, sweet, white)

Ground provisions (cassava, green banana, tania, dasheen, breadfruit, plantain, etc.)

Buckwheat (not related to wheat and not a grain but a pseudo grain) may not be tolerated by people with really sensitive GI tracts

DR. LISA'S NOTES

» You can't "moderate" yourself from generational illness toward exceptional health. You need to be steadfast and committed.
» Reactive gluten is found in wheat, barley, rye, and triticale, but also in spelt, farro, and kamut.
» The label "gluten-free" doesn't mean healthy.

WELLNESS PRESCRIPTION

» Have you been considering removing gluten and/or grain from your primary diet? Good! Within the next 24 hours, *take action.* Avoid bread, grain, and pasta. Instead, select items to incorporate into your meals from my list of delicious non-grain alternatives. Then use that momentum to build a lifestyle where you are FINE-ally free!

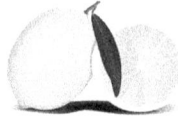

Chapter 9

FIBER-FILLED

*Don't play games with your health. The
system is rigged. You'll never win.*

Before boarding an early flight in Las Vegas to go back home, I wearily pulled out a packaged snack I got from the hotel room. Once on the flight, I tore the wrapper off the pecan bar and flipped the package over to read more. It said, "Half the sugar of an apple." Obviously, the manufacturers of the snack bar thought that was a great selling point to drive more sales of their product. But I was slightly annoyed by the statement.

No matter how much sugar an apple has, fresh fruit beats packaged food every time. Fresh fruits, including apples, offer a plethora of benefits since they also contain nutrients, minerals, antioxidants, and, of course, fiber.

For that reason, there are numerous benefits associated with including plants as part of every meal. Plants are fiber-filled! Unfortunately, ninety-five percent of Americans don't get enough fiber. That's astonishing since fiber is an essential part of nutrition and well-being. A lack of fiber can lead to inflammation and digestive issues, as well as poor digestive health.

Fiber is the roughage that comes from plants that cannot be digested by the human body. In fact, no animal—not even a cow or a goat—can digest cellulose, the main constituent of plant fiber. It just travels right through you, bringing tremendous benefits.

Fiber is naturally and easily found in fruits, vegetables, nuts, seeds, and legumes. The skin of fruits and vegetables is a great source of dietary fiber.

There are two types of fiber. They are classified according to whether they dissolve in water. *Soluble fiber* forms a dissolvable gel when mixed with water. It is useful in maintaining blood sugar control and reducing cholesterol. *Insoluble fiber*, however, does not form a gel when mixed with water and passes through the gastrointestinal tract mostly intact. Insoluble fiber is the part that comes out of the body as poop. Since both soluble and insoluble fiber have different functions in the body, we need both.

The sad truth is that only 5 percent of Americans get enough fiber. Most Americans only eat 10 to 15 grams of fiber per day when we actually need much more. Women younger than fifty need 25 grams of fiber, while men under age fifty need 38 grams. When it comes to the over-fifty crowd, women and men need a bit less—21 and 30 grams of fiber per day, respectively.

Besides keeping you regular and metabolically fit, fiber has a tremendous role in cancer prevention. Studies have shown that eating foods high in fiber have a protective effect, not only against colon cancer but also against ovarian cancer, breast cancer, and more. In fact, researchers have shown that women who eat high-fiber foods have had a reduction in breast cancer incidence compared to women who consumed less fiber. Fiber intake also decreases the risk of prostate cancer and coronary heart disease. This is one of the reasons you must strive to eat a variety of fruits and vegetables every day.

A RAINBOW OF FRUITS AND VEGETABLES

A rainbow of colors, including red, green, orange/yellow, and blue/purple, are super important when eating fruits and vegetables.

Not only will you get much needed vitamins, minerals, and phytonutrients by eating these colors, but it will also make it more likely that you'll reach your dietary fiber goals every day. Here's a breakdown of what "eating the rainbow" might look like. A quick heads up: We don't have to agree on what fruits and vegetables should be in which color categories—we'll leave that for art class. The point is to dive in.

Pink/Red

Apples, raspberries, guavas, pomegranates, peppers, strawberries, watermelons, cherries, red peppers, red chili peppers, tomatoes, cranberries, goji berries, blood oranges, dragon fruits, pink grapefruits, radishes, red beets

Orange/Yellow

Ackee, oranges, bananas, carrots, ground cherries, golden beets, passion fruits, papayas, mangos, squash, pumpkins, cantaloupes, nectarines, apricots, star fruits (carambola), peaches, kenips (genips), pineapples, lemons, sweet potatoes

Green

Apples, aloe, kale, spinach, broccoli, kiwi, zucchini, avocados, peppers, asparagus, peas, lima beans, green beans, Brussels sprouts, cabbage, celery, green grapes, pears, okra, cucumbers, green onions, honeydew melons

Blue/Purple

Blueberries, blackberries, eggplant, red grapes, plums, purple potatoes, red onions, red leaf kale, purple cabbage

White

Cassava (yams), coconut, soursop (guanábana), ginger, parsnips, sugar apples, breadfruit, dasheen, cauliflower, garlic, jicama, mushrooms, onions, cauliflower, potatoes, lychees, mangosteens

In addition, make sure to eat organic produce whenever possible. If they're edible and organic, you should always opt to leave the skins on fruits and vegetables. Just give them a good wash under fresh, running water first.

If you remove the skins from vegetables like carrots, only remove the thinnest layer. Packed with vitamins, nutrients, and fiber, those skins are good for you. God built the perfect package. Don't mess up a good thing.

As a matter of fact, eating the fiber-rich skin along with the fruit or vegetable helps slow down the absorption of sugar and reduces insulin spikes. That is a good thing since those spikes can lead to nutritional imbalance, inflammation, and chronic disease.

The following is a selection of produce with edible skins. While some of the fruits and vegetables on this list will be a no-brainer, others may be a surprise.

Again, when consuming the skins of fruits and vegetables, always make sure you source organic options and wash them thoroughly.

Produce with Edible Skins

Apples – Make sure to source organic apples, and don't throw away the skins.

Bananas – The skins are totally edible and contain lots of fiber. They can be cooked and used as a meat substitute in vegan dishes. You can also try blending the skins and including them in smoothies for extra fiber or using them as a tasty addition to any healthy muffin recipe.

Blueberries

Carrots – Save the carrot peeler for something else!

Cherries

Kiwis

Grapes

Lemons – Grate the skin to use as lemon zest. Just 1 tablespoon contains 9 percent of the daily recommended value of vitamin C.

Limes – Preferred as zest.

Mangoes – My kids wouldn't dare let this go to waste.

Melon – Yep, the rind is completely edible raw. You can also try eating it pickled or blended in fresh juice.

Oranges – Biting into an orange with the skin may give you a bad case of stomach cramps. Alternatively, you can try using some grated orange rind in your cooking or having some candied honey rind as a treat.

Peaches

Peppers – Peppers are fruits.

Plums

Strawberries

Tomatoes – I need to get this off my chest. Tomatoes are fruits. Whew! That feels better.

Potatoes

Sweet potatoes

Some high-fiber foods you can incorporate into your lifestyle are listed below. Note that this is not a complete list. Due to common food intolerances and GI disturbances, some items have been consequently left off.

High-Fiber Fruits, Vegetables, Nuts, and Seeds per Serving

Food Serving Size Fiber (in grams per serving)

Guava – 1 cup, 8.90 grams
Green peas (cooked) – 1 cup, 8.84 grams
Soursop – 1 cup, 7.40 grams
Gooseberries – 1 cup, 6.50 grams
Wild blueberries – 1 cup, 6.20 grams
Passion fruit – 1/4 cup, 6.10 grams
Pumpkin seeds – 1 ounce, 5.20 grams
Avocados – 1/2 cup, 5.00 grams
Grapefruit – 1 fruit, 5.00 grams
Quinoa (cooked) – 1 cup, 5.00 grams
Apple with skin – medium, 4.80 grams
Kale (cooked) – 1 cup, 4.70 grams
Coconut – 1 ounce, 4.60 grams
Chia seeds – 1 tablespoon, 4.10 grams
Pomegranate seeds – 1/2 cup, 4.00 grams
Papaya – 1 cup, 3.91 grams
Star fruit (carambola) – 1 cup, 3.70 grams
Almonds – 1 ounce, 3.50 grams
Prunes – 1/4 cup, 3.10 grams
Sunflower seeds – 1 ounce, 3.10 grams
Flaxseeds – 1 tablespoon, 2.80 grams
Sesame seeds – 1 tablespoon, 2.00 grams
Mangos – 3/4 cup, 2.00 grams

The More You Know, the More You Glow!

Do you know that baru nuts (a nut indigenous to South America) has the most fiber per serving than any other nut? At 5 grams per 30 gram serving, these nuts pack a powerful and nutritious punch.

DR. LISA'S NOTES

» Most people don't get enough fiber.
» No matter your food and dietary preferences, it's important that you eat a plethora of fresh and lightly cooked organic fruits and vegetables at every meal.

WELLNESS PRESCRIPTION

» In addition to eating fruits and vegetables, consider adding a fiber supplement free of artificial colors, flavors, and unnecessary sugars.

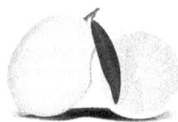

Chapter 10

BE PLANTIFUL!

What you like and what your body needs aren't always the same things. Learn to tell the difference, and adjust accordingly.

What you eat is important. A diet consisting of dunked, sugared, dipped, battered, genetically modified plants will do nothing positive for your health, even if they're 100 percent plant-based.

Eat more plants, but remember that paying attention to *how* those plants are prepared is also key. That means including fresh fruits, vegetables, herbs, roots, and shoots.

Plants contain powerful phytonutrients, enzymes, and antioxidants that are beneficial whether eaten raw or cooked. To get the most nutritional bang for your buck, you should enjoy a combination of both raw and cooked fruits and vegetables. When it comes to cooking those plants, lightly steamed vegetables are nutritionally preferred over boiled, while boiled is better than broiled, and broiled is favored over fried.

EAT PLANT-RICH, NOT PLANT-POOR

At the time of writing this book, I own a wellness website and have a growing social media presence. People often send me direct messages online with the assumption that I follow a plant-based diet. But here's the thing. You don't have to follow a plant-based diet to live plant-rich.

Part of being FINE is about eating plant-rich versus being plant-poor. If you're eating a vast array of brightly colored vegetables and fruits, as well as nuts and seeds with good fats and wild fish and pasture-raised meat, you're in the green zone. Notice I said "vegetables and fruits" versus "fruits and vegetables."

Often, it's not the lack of consumption of fruits that's the problem but the absence of a robust array of vegetables. As I mentioned in the previous chapter, eating the rainbow is key. An easy way to eat more colorful plants is by incorporating soups, stews, salads, and smoothies into your diet.

When it comes to making soup, you can get as simple or as complex as you like. In the spring and fall months, I prefer simple soups such as tomato red pepper soup, spicy butternut squash bisque, and carrot ginger soup. Once winter rolls around, it's time for chicken soup, beef soup, and stews. Stay away from flour, cheese, and cream-based soups. Instead, use ingredients such as sweet potatoes, parsnips, pumpkins, and squash to thicken your soup.

For a creamy soup without dairy, try adding coconut milk or macadamia nut milk. If you can tolerate beans, blend some cannellini beans to add that creamy texture that you crave.

Don't forget to add carrots, celery, mushrooms, kale, and your favorite vegetables and herbs.

Smoothies are also great. To make sure your smoothies aren't just a shot of sugar in a glass, add a cup or two of leafy greens such as spinach or kale to your fruits. Adding a spoonful of unsweetened almond butter is also a clean option for protein and a good source of fiber.

Salads are an easy way to pack lots of produce into your day. If you're keeping things FINE, here are some tips for your next salad. First, avoid cheese, croutons, and any cream-based dressings. With any dressing, you should be able to *see* the lettuce, greens, or produce. To make your own salad dressing at home, use one part vinegar or lemon juice, three parts olive oil, salt and pepper, and any fresh herbs or spices you like.

Here's a story: When I was sixteen, we went to visit my uncle on another island. His wife graciously welcomed us into their home with lunch and a freshly made salad. I don't remember everything that was on the menu, but I do remember that the salad dressing was homemade. It consisted of lemon juice, olive oil, and simple herbs. But to be honest, I wasn't as healthfully awakened as I am today. At the time, her efforts were grossly unappreciated on my teenage taste buds. Stories like this one make me laugh out loud today and reveal that growth is possible no matter where you are or where you've started.

PHYTO POWER

Eating plants is not optional when choosing a robust and healthy life. The consumption of certain plants has even been linked to the reduction of diseases and conditions such as cancer, hypertension, diabetes, high cholesterol, and more.

Depending on your wellness goals, you'll want to pay attention to which plants have the upper hand in fiber, antioxidants, vitamins, minerals, and other phytonutrients.

In addition, when deciding which fruits and vegetables to load up on, be sure to take into consideration your hemoglobin A1C, any existing disease states, inflammation, and allergies. For example, someone with diabetes or challenges pertaining to high blood sugar should not be drinking morning juices every day made solely from bananas, strawberries, and pineapples. Why not? While drinking fresh juice may be better than eating a donut for breakfast, the impact of drinking those peeled fruits with their small juiced particle sizes without the benefit of fiber from their skins can have an unwanted rapid and rising effect on blood sugar. Fiber in fruits and vegetables also has the added benefit of keeping you full.

By the way, just to be clear, I don't advocate that anyone subscribe to a fruit-juice-only routine regardless of perceived blood sugar control. As mentioned previously, a more favorable option is using a combination of fruits and vegetables, roots, and potentially some added protein for a nourishing drink with a plethora of health benefits.

The same thing goes for smoothies. Packing smoothies with things such as greens, veggies, fiber, and clean protein, in addition to your desired fruit, is one of the keys to living life the FINE way.

Favorite Smoothie Blend-Ins

Add these to any of your smoothies for a big nutritional impact.

Bee pollen
Bone broth powder

Cinnamon
Chia seeds
Chlorella
Clean protein powder
Collagen
Kale
Fiber
Flax seeds
Ginger
Matcha powder
Spinach
Spirulina
Turmeric
Unsweetened nut butter
Wheatgrass (naturally gluten-free since it is grown and harvested without seeds)

KNOW YOUR FRUITS

As we delve more deeply, the biology nerd in me has to bring up a very important point regarding the difference between fruits and vegetables. If I don't, memories of undergraduate classes in plant physiology and terrestrial plant biology will haunt me greatly, and I'm sure none of us want that.

It's occurred to me that most people don't know the difference between fruits and vegetables. Several fruits are routinely called vegetables, and even some grains are often misclassified as vegetables too.

It's a whole mess. It's no wonder the body is so confused. Most people don't even know what they're eating! So let's start here. Fruits don't have to be sweet in the general sense. Botanically, to be classified as a fruit, the plant part must contain seeds. That's because fruits are the ripened ovary of the plant. The contents of that ripened ovary are known as seeds. Fruits can further be classified as grains or even squash.

Here's a list of fruits that are often (inaccurately) referred to as vegetables.

Avocados
Cucumbers
Eggplant

Okra
Peppers
Pumpkins
Tomatoes

Notice that the definition for fruit doesn't take into consideration how you cook the plant or what you eat it with. What matters is the internal structure. And if you're eating the ripened ovary of a plant, you're eating a fruit.

For the purposes of this book, your morning meal (often referred to as breakfast) should not consist of just fruits. However, fruits can be combined with protein, vegetables, quality fats (such as ghee, coconut oil, avocado oil, and olive oil), roots, shoots, and pseudograins for a sensible meal.

KNOW YOUR VEGETABLES

A vegetable is any edible part of a plant—roots, stems, leaves, flowers, bark, or the entire plant. Vegetables are naturally low in sugar and high in vitamins, minerals, antioxidants, and fiber. Some of the healthiest vegetables are cruciferous in nature.

Cruciferous vegetables are a group of low-calorie, edible plants that are rich in nutrients and vitamins. The reason these plants are known by the name cruciferous is because they possess four petaled flowers that look like a cross.

It's as if God himself has given a divine sign about what to eat.

Cruciferous vegetables are noted to be particularly high in vitamins and minerals, and contain compounds known as glucosinolates that are associated with fighting and reducing cancer. Part of the reason cruciferous vegetables are so special is the abundance of vitamins and minerals such as vitamins A, C, and folate. These vegetables are also a great source of dietary fiber.

Vegetables in the cruciferous family include the following:

Arugula
Bok choy
Broccoli
Broccoli rabe

Broccolini
Brussels sprouts
Cabbage
Cauliflower
Chard
Chinese cabbage
Collard greens
Daikon
Horseradish
Kale
Kohlrabi
Mustard greens
Radishes
Romanesco
Rutabaga
Turnips
Turnip greens
Wasabi
Watercress

Sulforaphane, a compound rich in sulfur, is found in cruciferous vegetables and has a direct effect on limiting stress and inflammation caused by oxidation in the body. That happens through a pathway known as NrF2. It's this chronic inflammation and added stress that underlie neurodegenerative diseases such as Parkinson's, Alzheimer's, Huntington's disease, and other brain and spinal cord diseases. Mitochondrial decline is also implicated.

This is important because with the way things are going, neurodegenerative diseases are now one of the biggest threats to healthy aging.

Targeting the NrF2 pathway provides the protection and detoxification needed to reduce this added stress and disease. In addition, several studies point to slowed tumor growth and the blocking of DNA mutation, which makes cruciferous vegetables a powerful part of the prevention and treatment of various cancers.

Here's the bottom line. I'm not going to harp on you about eating your Brussels sprouts. But if you're not eating Brussels sprouts, I hope you're eating lots of kale, broccoli, cabbage, daikon radishes, and other cruciferous vegetables to fill the gap.

You should always include plants in your diet, no matter what "lifestyle" you follow. They should not be only processed plants that were made to act or taste like the foods you used to eat, but real plants—the stuff you can still recognize when you eat it. When you eat plants this way, you won't have to ask, "What's this made of?" because the answer will be abundantly clear. That's not to say that plants formed into a burger, a chip, or a dip cannot be enjoyed. It does mean that they should be eaten in addition to less processed vegetables as part of a healthy diet.

If you're eating unhealthy, plant-based versions of everything you used to eat, there could be a problem.

Let's be clear. Plant-based cream cheese, vegan burgers, and vegan hotdogs are still processed foods. You can certainly enjoy them, but don't get stuck in the mindset that they are healthy foods. They should not be the majority of your diet.

The point is to eat more quality produce, herbs, nuts, and seeds. If you're determined to live a FINE life, then non-GMO vegetables and fruits should be part of every meal.

Remember, Oreos are technically vegan! So food labels are not what make people healthy. Knowing how to eat, when to eat, what to eat, and why you eat is important. Focusing on whether the food you're eating is restorative versus depletive is a better indicator of good health than any dietary labels you impose on yourself.

Living a plant-rich life means that every meal (not including snacks) should involve eating plants. It's just that simple. Eat fresh plants, steamed plants, pureed plants, blended plants, and baked or roasted plants. Eat plants at every meal along with whatever else you're eating. Some of those plants you eat should also be raw.

Being plantiful means focusing on vegetables, including spinach, kale, chard, mushrooms, zucchini, cauliflower, lettuce, green beans, and blue potatoes, and enjoying fruits in their whole form as a major part of the diet. Pasture-raised meats, grass-fed beef, and wild fish are tasty alongside and can be enjoyed for filling, healthy, and satisfying meals.

Eating plantifully is for everyone. The best part is that you don't have to be plant-based to enjoy it. Taking a look through human history, we know that we've been eating plants for several millennia.

As hunter-gatherers, we received much of our nourishment from grasses, tubers, nuts, seeds, and foraging. The ability to hunt large animals didn't come until later and the agricultural period not until long after that. Eating a plant-rich diet is for everyone. That includes those who enjoy a juicy T-bone steak with steamed kale and an unloaded baked sweet potato on the side.

Important to Note

If you're suffering from digestive issues such as IBS, a plate filled with cruciferous vegetables may be the *last* thing you want to eat due to the potential of gastric distress. However, since IBS can be caused by anything from emotional stress to imbalances of the gut microbiome, food intolerances, and more, it's important to work with a naturopath to get to the bottom of what's causing your symptoms and the best way to heal.

For some, things such as consistent exercise, mindful practices, probiotics, and herbal botanicals may be just what you need to get relief and return to eating a diverse array of vegetables for abundant health.

A DAY OF EATING PLANTIFUL

Are you an omnivore who wants to eat more plants to Be FINE? Here's what a day of eating plantiful can look like for you.

First meal: A bowl of cooked quinoa enveloped by almond milk and topped with organic blueberries and walnuts, along with two boiled eggs.

Second meal: Stir-fried cauliflower rice with vegetables such as peppers, onions, garlic, ginger, mushrooms, and broccoli, topped with wild salmon or other clean protein of choice.

Third meal: Grilled chicken breasts or grass-fed beef with baked sweet potato and sautéed lemon kale.

DR. LISA'S NOTES

» Eating more plants is not reserved for a certain group of indi-viduals—it's for everyone, including you.
» Focusing on whether the food you're eating is restorative or deple-tive is a better indicator of good health than any dietary labels you impose on yourself.
» A group of vegetables called the cruciferous family contains some of the most powerful phytonutrients that fight inflammation and limit disease.

WELLNESS PRESCRIPTION

» Include at least three servings of cruciferous vegetables in your meal plan this week.

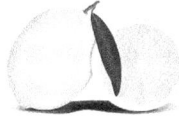

Chapter 11

OH, SUGAR SUGAR!

If your list of "can'ts" is bigger than your list of "cans," then you're not looking for wellness; you're looking for convenience.

Okay, we're here—the part of the book you desperately need to read to liberate yourself fully and freely.

Just kidding. That's actually the entire book.

But this part will profoundly change the way you think about fat and sugar. The fat-free fallacy is the mistaken belief that fat is *bad* and grains (especially things such as whole grains, wheat bread, oats, etc.) are *good.*

Uncomfortable yet?

Let's dive in.

There are three major nutritional macromolecules: fat, carbohydrates, and protein. Over the past fifty years, one macromolecule has been pegged as the "bad guy."

Called out.

Dragged out.

Written up and plastered all over TV and the media.

I won't go into all the details, but this started sometime in the 1960s when the American Health Association (AHA) came out with a statement that saturated fat was very bad and that limiting all dietary fats was a good thing to do. Those fats were thought to be a cause of heart disease, and they recommended eating less than 300 mg of fat per day.

That helped set the tone for other organizations such as the United States Department of Agriculture (USDA) to come up with the food pyramid, which essentially guided Americans on what and how to eat.

This guidance leaned heavily on eating more carbohydrates and less meats and fats. The foundation of the pyramid was carbohydrates: bread, pasta, crackers, and cereal. Everyone from professional athletes to animated bees and tigers echoed the sentiments of eating a "heart-healthy" breakfast. A typical heart-healthy breakfast included a bowl of store-bought cereal or oatmeal, toast, and a glass of orange juice.

The big problem with this approach is that fats are very satisfying to consume and help make you feel full. Aside from the fearmongering about cholesterol, fats are a good and necessary part of the human diet.

So how did the manufacturers of processed foods compensate for the removal of fat?

They loaded their products with sugar in all its forms, and particularly corn syrup.

It was a carb and sugar lover's dream. Eventually, there would be symbols on everything from sugary cereals to snack bars about what to eat. They were endorsed, after all. At the same time, people were led to believe that limiting fats and protein (no matter their source) was a good idea.

This advice led to centripetal obesity (fat around the stomach and midsection) and the renaming of adult-onset diabetes to merely type 2 diabetes (since children were now presenting with the disease). For the first time in history, a generation of children are not outliving their parents. Low-fat and no-fat foods took over the grocery store shelves and ad slots on television.

Today, it's not out of the ordinary to see cookies, snack bars, and even brightly colored gummy snacks proudly displaying fat-free labels. In the place of fat, you'll find artificial colors, flavors, and more sugar and carbohydrates than ever before. The decoded message: fat is out; sugar and carbs are in.

This archaic advice is why belly bulge is such an issue. The battle of the bulge is not just a nuisance, but wider waist lines can put you at greater risk for cardiovascular disease. Actually, waist to hip circumference is even more important than BMI in predicting cardiovascular risk. Limit refined sugars, refrain from grains, follow a consistent exercise regimen, and your body will be more than happy to give you what you want and need. Following two out of three things just won't cut it. As a matter of fact, what worked at age twenty-five won't work at thirty-five, forty-five, fifty-five, or sixty-five. So you might as well adapt and lean into change now. Your body is capable of amazing things.

Faulty advice about fats and sugars explains why 100 million Americans have fatty liver disease, about 40 million Americans suffer from type 2 diabetes, and 88 million Americans (one in three) are pre-diabetic.

After my graduate studies, I eagerly took part in a diabetes management program. Hoping to make a difference in the diabetes community, other healthcare providers and I went out into minority communities and asked questions about smoking cessation, alcohol consumption, and prescription medication compliance.

Diet was never a factor.

Therein lies the problem: insulin resistance that has been linked to everything from diabetes, coronary heart disease (CHD), cancer, dyslipidemia (high cholesterol), polycystic ovarian syndrome (PCOS), and hypertension has everything to do with diet.

It's not the fat that is the primary issue but the massive amounts of carbohydrates and . . . well . . . ummm, I'll let you guess . . .

SUGAR.

SWEET THING

You: "I just have a sweet tooth!"

Your body: "No, you're a sugar addict."

When a person ingests fat, barely any change to their fasting blood sugar levels takes place. Protein has a bit more of an effect on blood sugar levels, with carbohydrates having the biggest effect of all the macromolecules. Whether you're diabetic or not, fasting blood glucose is a really important aspect of healthy aging, unwanted weight gain, and disease prevention. What I'm saying is that fat is not enemy number one. The wrong type of carbohydrates paired with the wrong fats is.

Now this is not to say that a bunless cheeseburger with a side of lard should be your next power meal. But knowing what type of foods increase blood sugar and the type of impact you can expect from them is certainly part of the equation.

GLYCEMIC INDEX

This brings us to the concept of glycemic index. You may be familiar with high-carb, low-carb, high-sugar, and low-sugar foods, but do you know what the glycemic index is?

Glycemic index (GI) is a way to track how quickly food is broken down into glucose, which your body uses for fuel. The values for glycemic index range from 0 to 100 with the GI of glucose tracking in at 100.

When you're planning meals, take into consideration which ingredients are inflammatory versus non-inflammatory, but also pay attention to the glycemic index of those foods. Fruits such as pineapples, watermelons, and ripe bananas are naturally high in sugar, which your body quickly digests. As a result, these foods have a moderate to high glycemic index. Since fruits also contain high amounts of fiber (which slows the release of sugar), minerals, and vitamins, the effect on blood sugar is more minimal than other high glycemic foods.

Similarly, pairing moderate to high glycemic index foods with low glycemic index foods can lower the overall impact on blood sugar by decreasing the total glycemic index for the entire meal. As you may expect, the highest glycemic index foods are also the ones with the biggest fan clubs. They include foods such as white rice, fries, potato chips, cookies, cake, crackers, brown and white bread, flavored yogurt, and instant oatmeal. Using this principle as a guide, it would be wiser to have a bowl of flaxseed cereal for breakfast topped with blueberries and walnuts than to have a bowl of instant oatmeal topped with sliced bananas and drizzled with honey.

While both may sound like equally good choices for a healthy breakfast, your body doesn't process those meals the same way. The oatmeal will result in a quick rise of blood sugar levels, while the flaxseed yields a more stable and less erratic glucose sugar response.

Another healthy and more insulin-resistant option is eggs, smoked salmon, and some fresh greens. This type of meal will keep you fuller longer without unpredictable insulin spikes and crashes.

Don't use this information as a permission slip to gorge yourself on just any low glycemic foods. After all, some low glycemic foods are incredibly unhealthy—Snickers bars have a glycemic index of 43, and Nutella spread has a glycemic index of 33. Both of these foods are addicting and high in sugar and calories. Not only will overindulging in these foods spike your blood sugar, but calories, sugar content, and the presence of unhealthy fats add to inflammation and can have devastating effects on your health.

Glycemic Index Scale

Low glycemic index foods – less than 55
Medium glycemic index foods – 56–69
High glycemic index foods – 70 or higher

While the glycemic index is a powerful tool, it's just one of many variables that should be considered in crafting a FINE meal. Protein, fiber, nutrient content, and fat should be used in concert to minimize exaggerated insulin spikes. Not only will meals with good fats keep blood sugar levels stable, but incorporating those fats into meals will keep you feeling fuller longer.

When a food is classified as high glycemic, it means it is quickly broken down, digested, and absorbed by the body for energy. A sharp spike in blood sugar is the result. That causes the pancreas to release insulin. If cells start to absorb the sugar too quickly, a rapid fall in blood sugar can ensue, resulting in frequent hunger and less time between meals.

Insulin release causes the uptake of sugar to muscle, liver, and fat cells. The food input is used as energy, and any excess sugar is stored as fat in the liver. This fat can travel to the bloodstream and cause issues with triglycerides and cholesterol, leading to cardiovascular disease. The result is a roller coaster of insulin surges and plummets.

A continuous presence of carbohydrates prevents the body from using its own fat as fuel. In the meantime, since insulin acts as a fat storage hormone, high insulin levels result in extra sugars being stored as fat. Weight gain is the result. That is especially true around the liver and gut area, and it is the reason so many people have a problem with excess belly fat.

Eventually, cells become less sensitive to insulin. The resulting buildup of sugar in the blood feeds viruses and bacteria, and can even cause nerve damage.

In people who don't eat excess carbohydrates and sugar, the body turns to burning fat (either fat in the diet or the body's fat stores) for energy. Essentially, your body becomes a fat-burning, belly-blasting machine. Sounds efficient, right?

It's important to note that both carbohydrates and fat can be burned for energy. Carbohydrates provide more quick energy that needs to be refueled often, while fats provide more slow energy that is more efficient.

It's not that you should eliminate carbohydrates from your diet entirely, The body needs carbs, protein, and fat to function effectively. You just need to focus on eating the right types of non-refined carbs for fuel.

Examples of FINE Carbs:

Beans (if tolerated)
Breadfruit
Buckwheat (if tolerated)
Fruits (pay attention to glycemic index)
Green bananas
Parsnips
Pumpkins
Purple potatoes
Quinoa
Sweet potatoes

If you struggle with unwanted weight gain, it's likely that you're eating too many of the wrong types of carbohydrates and sugars. I once heard a woman say that all she has to do is smell bread and she gains weight. Obviously she was joking, but you can sense how frustrating and difficult that must be. Not only is her body storing much of the energy she consumes as fat, but her body is not effectively using fat as fuel.

THE MANY FORMS OF SUGAR

Sugar is wreaking absolute havoc on the health of millions of people every day.

And while you may think you know when you're eating sugar, do you *really* know?

Sugar is hidden in places you wouldn't even expect, including in 74 percent of packaged foods. If you're eating candy or donuts, you definitely expect there to be some sugar. But would you expect there to be sugar in salad dressing, pasta sauce, bread, bacon, or condiments?

More Foods with Hidden Sugar

Applesauce and fruit purees
Baking mixes
Breakfast cereals
Deli and cured meats

Diet foods
Juices
Flavored waters
Granola bars
Oatmeal packets
Potato chips
Pizza sauce
Trail mix
Vitamins and supplements
Yogurt

Do you know that there are more than 50 names for sugar? It's all part of the sneaky tricks that food companies use so you really don't know what you're getting or eating. While not all sugars are created equal, it's a good idea to keep this list in mind when you're reading food labels.

Other Names for the Sweet Stuff

Agave syrup or nectar
Barbados sugar
Barley malt
Beet sugar
Blackstrap molasses
Brown sugar
Brown rice syrup
Buttered sugar or buttercream
Cane sugar
Caramel
Carob syrup
Castor sugar
Coconut sugar
Confectioner's sugar (powdered sugar)
Corn syrup
Crystalline fructose
Date sugar
Date syrup
Demerara sugar
Dextrose
Dextrin
Diastatic malt

Ethyl maltol
Evaporated cane juice
Florida crystals
Fruit syrup
Fruit syrup concentrate
Fructose
Galactose
Golden sugar
Glucose syrup solids
Grape sugar
High fructose corn syrup (HFCS)
Honey
Icing sugar
Invert sugar
Lactose
Liquid syrup
Maple syrup
Maltodextrin
Maltose
Malt syrup
Maple syrup
Muscovado sugar
Panela sugar
Raw sugar
Refiner's syrup
Rice syrup
Simple syrup
Sorghum syrup
Sugar (granulated or table)
Sucanat
Sucrose
Treacle
Turbinado sugar
Yellow sugar

This list was provided not to intimidate but to empower you through education versus trepidation. All sugars are not created equal, of course. But you owe it to yourself to know what you're eating. In the next chapter, we'll talk about some of those differences and smart sugar selection (SSS).

Which of These Describe You?

"I can't quit sugar."

"I don't have a problem with sugar. I'm a big bread person."

"I have a major sweet tooth."

"I just have to have a little something sweet after every meal."

"I don't eat sugar. Period. Coffee is my jam: vanilla latte with soy milk and eight pumps of vanilla and extra caramel drizzle."

"I've never liked sugar. I don't even eat cake! My diet is pretty good actually. For example, today for breakfast I had a bowl of Rice Krispies with bananas and almond milk. For lunch I had a vegetable rice noodle bowl. For dinner I had chicken fried rice followed by a small serving of rice pudding for dessert."

Newsflash: All these scenarios demonstrate a huge problem with sugar!

Sweet Tricks They Play

Food companies are really sneaky about the "sweet tricks" they play. For example, always remember that all forms of sugar are "natural" food products. If you see a food label that proclaims the product is "all natural—no artificial ingredients," rest assured it can still contain plenty of sugar.

Here's another trick that food companies use and why it's one of the worst sugars you can consume.

You've heard of high fructose corn syrup (HFCS), right? You may have heard that HFCS is not good for you, but do you know why?

HFCS is found in thousands of products, from salad dressings to soft drinks, snacks, and desserts. HFCS can also be very detrimental to your health.

Shhh . . . they don't want you to know!

HFCS alters hundreds of genes in the brain and prevents you from recognizing cues that you're full. Literally, HFCS desensitizes the receptors in the brain that let you know when to stop eating. So you keep eating and feel like you can't get enough of your favorite snack foods and beverages. Meanwhile, it's more than about willpower because your brain is literally under submissive attack.

That's why fueling with the right kinds of foods and understanding why you should eat or not eat those foods are so vital.

But overeating is not the only issue here. HFCS can also lead to diabetes, obesity, visceral fat, fatty liver disease, chronic illness, and more.

Now that you know, feel free to do something about it.

Am I telling you that you should avoid all sugar for the rest of eternity? If you're addicted, that is certainly an individual consideration that everyone should make. Under most circumstances, I believe that education and mindful consumption is warranted.

In addition, once you start consistently fueling your body with the right kinds of foods, you'll find that you just won't want to eat the same amounts of sugar you've been used to. Give yourself ninety days to revamp those taste buds, and watch how the cookie crumbles . . . literally.

Smart Sugar Selection: This or That

I don't want to "sugarcoat" things, but I'm not a big fan of sugar substitutes. If you are limiting or avoiding refined sugar, you can use other options to get to the sweet side. On the occasions when you do have some sugar, choose smart, and choose simply.

Sugar Alcohols

Sugar alcohols have gone mainstream with the explosion of new, trendy diets. Examples of sugar alcohols include erythritol, maltitol, sorbitol, and xylitol. While they're not technically considered artificial sweeteners since they are found naturally in fruits and vegetables, sugar alcohols in your food were likely produced industrially.

Sugar alcohols are produced from carbohydrate products such as glucose through fermentation. Since sugar alcohols are low glycemic, low-calorie, and don't spike blood sugar, they have found favor in the "healthy diet" industry. So you'll see them in everything from wraps to puddings, drinks, chewing gum, and more.

So far, the overconsumption of sugar alcohols such as erythritol has been linked to flatulence, diarrhea, irritable bowel syndrome, and increased cardiovascular risk. Does that mean there are other long-term consequences of habitual sugar alcohol consumption that we don't yet know?

Possibly.

In the early 1930s and 1940s, there wasn't yet a clear link between cigarette smoking and cancer. So the tobacco industry hired medical professionals such as doctors to promote smoking cigarettes. They went as far as to say that doctors preferred smoking one brand of cigarettes over another.

Seems preposterous, right?

What I'm saying is, if you're solely waiting for the medical community to tell you what's good or bad for you, you're not leading with the right compass.

By the way, do you think the practice of paid medical endorsements by trusted medical professionals is always in your best interest?

I'll let you figure that one out.

Choose Smart

Few foods need to have refined sugar in them. Some easy ways to minimize the sugar in your diet is by omitting soft drinks, packaged juices, boxed cereals, and removing any sweeteners from hot beverages such as coffee and tea. In addition, reducing your reliance on packaged foods will greatly reduce your daily sugar intake.

Mindless snacking is another culprit of untamed sugar levels. Eating foods at mealtime that are high in quality protein, fiber, vitamins, and minerals will naturally diminish those sugar cravings.

Next, make sugar easily trackable. If you are not consuming erroneous sugars from other sources such as cold and hot beverages, cereals, packaged foods, and mindless snacking, it's easier to track sugar and stay on target.

Choose Simply

When I say choose simply, I mean to choose sweeteners made from plants versus those made by labs.

Pureed bananas, unsweetened applesauce, organic date puree or date syrup, wild honey, blackstrap molasses, and coconut sugar are acceptable options. While these natural sweeteners still contain sugar, they also contain vitamins and minerals that make them a better choice than white sugar or HFCS.

Blackstrap Molasses

Blackstrap molasses is the last byproduct of sugar production. The extraction process of sugar from the sugar cane results in three types of molasses. The sugar cane can grow roots up to fifteen feet deep. That in part is why blackstrap molasses is so nutritious. The roots go deep into the rich soil and carry those benefits to the resulting sweet sap.

The various types of molasses are identified by their dark color and viscosity after each round of extraction. Regular molasses is produced during phases one and two of boiling. Those products are light and dark molasses, respectively.

Blackstrap molasses is produced during the final stage of boiling. This molasses is the thickest and darkest in color, and has the most nutritional value.

Blackstrap molasses is much more nutritious than refined sugar. The iron content alone makes it worth a try. Just one tablespoon of blackstrap molasses has 20 percent of your daily value of iron.

It's also packed with magnesium, phosphorus, calcium, potassium, and vitamin B. The sticky sap also has a high amount of antioxidants and contains no artificial preservatives.

Maple Syrup

Another viable option you can consider is maple syrup. By no means is using maple syrup a panacea for a sugar addiction, but it does have some benefits over cane sugar.

Unlike table sugar or something like high fructose corn syrup, maple syrup contains vitamins and minerals, including vitamin B, folic acid, manganese, potassium, and more. These vitamins and minerals slow the absorption of the natural sweetener and have tremendous benefits.

Of course, everyone can make their own dietary decisions, but the point is to focus on "clean" foods that have high nutritional value and low glycemic and inflammatory impacts.

When it comes to sugar, what I've found is that it's not one ingredient that's the issue but several things combined. Foundational lifestyle choices paired with the never-ending access to carbs and grains, a lack of exercise, and nutrient-deficient foods are also paramount considerations.

When maple syrup is paired with an ingredient such as flaxseed, one of the most nutritionally dense, high-fiber foods, the blood sugar response will be more controlled and less sporadic than when eating carbs loaded with table sugar or HFCS.

This is the case with one of my most popular recipes—flaxseed quinoa porridge. The porridge is paired with low glycemic fruits such as blueberries. Walnuts can also be added as a crunchy topper. Walnuts have healthy fats and help slow the absorption of the sugar in the recipe.

Monk Fruit

Monk fruit, also known as *lo han guo*, is a fruit native to China. Once dried, this fruit is utilized as monk fruit sweetener. Monk fruit is much sweeter than sugar, has no calories or carbs, and is said to not raise blood sugar.

Stevia

While stevia sweetener is derived from the leaves of the stevia plant, there can be drawbacks, and we still have a lot to learn. If you choose to use stevia, opt for organic forms as pure liquid or pure organic powder. One of the issues with stevia is the possibility of counterfeit products. In addition, other artificial sweeteners have been found in manufactured stevia products, which may actually cause more harm than good.

We've now come to the end of the chapter. As you mind your sugar and carbs, be sure to add more protein and fiber, and increase your exercising too.

DR. LISA'S NOTES

» Food manufacturers hide sugar in all types of foods, using a variety of names.
» One of the most devastating of these sugars is high fructose corn syrup (HFCS).
» When you eat high fructose corn syrup, it interferes with a pathway in the brain that lets you know when you're full.

WELLNESS PRESCRIPTION

» Do an inventory of packaged foods in your home, and look for hidden sugars where they should not be. Of course, you'd expect to find maple syrup in 100 percent maple syrup (delicious when poured on grain-free pancakes, by the way), but it may come as a surprise to find sugar in things such as condiments or your favorite "healthy" hot cereal.

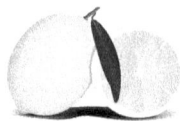

Chapter 12

BIG FAT LIES

Love yourself enough that you're willing to push through the discomfort to get to the life-changing part of your life.

As it turns out, sugar is not the only culprit standing between you and being FINE. Fat is also a concern, but it's not what you think. Unlike what you may have heard, all fat is not created equal. And being fat-free is absolutely not the way to be healthy.

The types of fats you consume, however, are a huge consideration. And let me tell you, too many people are eating the wrong types of fat.

Fortunately, the human body produces most of the fats you need, but there are two main fatty acids it cannot produce. These fats are omega-6 and omega-3, and they can only be obtained through exogenous sources in the diet.

While both of these fatty acids are needed for growth, development, and cell physiology, it's the imbalance of omega-6 fats between the two that can have devastating effects. Omega-6 fats such as linoleic acid (LA), a type of omega-6 fat, is found in seed oils, vegetable oils, and processed foods. Excess LA plays a role in inflammation and chronic diseases such as diabetes, heart disease, cancer, and dementia. Due to its use in many processed foods, the amount of LA has dramatically increased in the Western diet over the last few decades. As a result, the average person gets more than enough. These fats are also found in high-grain diets, and too much can be a significant cause of inflammation. If not balanced with healthy omega-3 fats, omega-6 fats can cause serious health concerns.

Alternatively, omega-3 fats are powerful tools in the fight against disease prevention, and they support healthy aging. There are three types of omega-3 fats.

Eicosapentaenoic acid (EPA) and docosahexaenoic acid (DHA) are both sourced naturally, mainly from wild fatty fish such as salmon, mackerel, sardines, herring, and trout. Alpha-linoleic acid (ALA), the most common omega-3, is found in foods such as walnuts, chia seeds, flax seeds, and seaweed.

The benefits of these fats include brain health, heart health, improvement of mood disorders, brain cognition, and more. But when it comes to the delicate balance between these two categories of omega-3 and omega-6 fats, there are several problems.

A major contributor to the overwhelming amount of omega-6 fats is the ingestion of seed oils. These are specific vegetable oils that come from the seeds of plants. They include corn oil, soybean oil, peanut oil, safflower oil, canola oil, peanut oil, and palm oil. When seed oils are consumed, your body breaks them down into harmful free radicals, which causes devastating oxidative damage and stress.

Seed oils are found in almost every processed food you can think of, including sauces, dressings, packaged nuts, snack foods, and, of course, fried foods. Grain-fed chicken, beef, and pork are other sources of heavily weighted omega-6 fats. Hence, organic pasture-raised chicken, grass-fed beef, and lamb are more suitable options.

Now that you know some sources of omega-6 fats, the point is to limit processed omega-6 fats and increase your level of omega-3 fats as much as possible.

Most people don't get enough omega-3 in their diet. And even when omega-3s are ingested, the ratio of omega-3 to omega-6 fatty acids is disproportionate, with omega-3 fats lagging far behind.

One way to get more omega-3 fats in your diet is by eating more wild-caught fatty fish such as salmon and mackerel. My in-laws bought fish from the same local fisherman for 45 years before he recently retired. Talk about getting your food from the source!

Sadly, the majority of fish sold in big supermarkets is mislabeled or fraudulent, so even when you think you're buying wild fish, you may not be getting the real thing. Selling mislabeled fish is big business!

The good news is that there are some readily accessible areas where you can easily make an impactful change. Omitting seed oils during cooking is one such area. Reducing processed foods is another. Instead of using seed oils, transition to other oils such as olive oil, avocado oil, and coconut oil. For salads and dressings, walnut oil and pure extra virgin olive oil are great options. Interestingly, chia seed oil is a great source of omega-3 fats and doesn't have the same negative effect of the seed oils we just discussed.

SWEET DECEIT

One of the biggest misconceptions about aging is that it has more to do with genes (what you can't control) and less to do with habits (what you can control), and I'm here to debunk this myth. Food, lifestyle habits, exercise, and appropriate nutrients weigh more heavily than what is reflected in your gene pool.

In fact, one of the biggest culprits of unhealthy aging is sugar. Specifically, the presence of advanced glycation end products, appropriately shortened to AGEs, is a major concern.

Also known as glycotoxins, AGEs are substances formed when certain protein or fat products are connected with sugar in the bloodstream. That causes a process known as glycation. The excess sugars, in combination with processed fats, are damaging to the skin and the body. They promote premature aging and harmful diseases. In the skin, these end products attach to collagen and make the skin less firm, lose its elasticity, and encourage wrinkles.

In other parts of the body, high AGEs lead to chronic illness such as heart disease, Alzheimer's, diabetes, high blood pressure, and increased inflammation, and it has been linked to cancer. To limit AGEs, a diet low in sugar is extremely important. In addition, foods and meats cooked at high dry temperatures, fried foods, and processed foods increase the production of AGEs.

While limiting the amount of sugar and reducing processed foods can have a significant impact, choosing the right method of cooking is also very important. Generally speaking, cooking methods that rely on low, slow, and moist heat are better than methods that rely on dry, high, and quick heat. These healthier methods of cooking include *sous vide*, slow cooking, and pressure cooking.

Not to be a killjoy, but barbecued and fried foods are generally prepared using high, dry heat. As such, if you're going to partake, I highly recommend limiting your intake and pairing such meats with natural AGE fighters such as cruciferous vegetables, seasonal produce, and wild or harvested mushrooms.

Fake Olive Oyl–I Mean, Olive Oil

Do you remember Popeye the Sailor Man cartoons? The animated character first came out in a cartoon strip in the 1920s and later became a televised cartoon series. While many parents gushed over the genius of an animated cartoon character getting super-strength powers from eating spinach, there's another superfood mentioned in this cartoon that you may have missed.

Olive oil.

Olive Oyl was Popeye's girlfriend. The pure, perhaps unintentional genius of this is that leafy green vegetables such as spinach contain fat-soluble vitamins A, D, E, and K. Fat-soluble vitamins are better absorbed with the addition of fats such as—you guessed it, olive oil.

In other words, olive oil enhances the bioavailability (what our body can use) of the vitamins in spinach. Did the creators of Popeye give much thought to the health benefits of eating spinach with olive oil when they were writing this cartoon? I have no idea. But I'd like to think they did.

Besides fat soluble vitamins, olive oil also contains linoleic acid (LA). The amount of LA is minimal when compared to processed oils such as safflower, canola, soybean, and peanut oils. Olive oil also contains a lot of healthy fats and antioxidants such as oleic acid and polyphenols.

Do you remember when I told you that you had to be a food detective? Well, up to 80 percent of olive oil sold in grocery stores is fraudulent. Unfortunately, many of the bad brands are thinned out with cheaper inflammatory seed oils. Like mislabeled fish, counterfeit olive oil is big business!

On a trip to South Africa years ago, I distinctly remember realizing that I had unknowingly been using counterfeit olive oil for years. I dipped my bread in the authentic golden juice and took a bite. The fruity notes followed by a light pepper note hit the back of my tongue right away. I still remember the gut-wrenching feeling of realizing I had been duped for all those years.

Here are some shopping tips to increase the chances that you'll be buying real olive oil on your next grocery trip.

Pay attention to how the olive oil is bottled. Olive oil should be packaged in glass, not plastic bottles. Olive oil bottled in dark, opaque bottles will stay fresh and minimize oxidation.

Stamps of third-party certification can also be helpful. In particular, the California Olive Oil Council (COOC) and the European Union's Protected Designation of Origin (PDO) are some names and designations to look for.

Only buy olive oil that says "extra virgin" on the bottle. Although not guaranteed, labels that say only "olive oil," "light olive oil," or "pure" are not good signs of authenticity.

Real extra virgin olive oil can vary in taste, but generally grassy, fruity, and peppery notes are good signs.

True extra virgin oil is not cheap. The best olive oil is pressed from younger olives to maximize polyphenol content. These young olives are unripe and have less juice per press. Hence, you need more olives to make a batch of good olive oil. That increases the price of the oil.

Olives, and thus olive oil, have been around for thousands of years. Olive oil is mentioned in the Bible, and it is well-known that Queen Cleopatra used olive oil as part of her beauty and wellness regimen. You can use olive oil topically by adding it to your favorite lotions, facial products, and conditioners, or you can use it by itself.

In addition, olive oil is beneficial when taken as a wellness shot. Do you know that olives are actually fruits? (There's a seed inside!) So when you consume olive oil, you are actually drinking fruit juice.

Some of the benefits of drinking olive oil include reduced inflammation, improved cardiovascular health, digestive health, and healthier skin and hair. People of the Mediterranean region have touted the benefits of drinking olive oil for centuries, even drinking one-fourth cup in the morning upon awakening. A FINE life includes using healthy fats such as olive oil to promote optimal wellness and well-being.

EGGS-ACTLY MY POINT

In 1968, as part of its anti-fat campaign, the American Health Association came out with guidance that Americans should eat no more than three whole egg yolks per week in order to lower cholesterol and reduce the chance of heart disease. Sometime after that, eating egg whites (no yolks) became a thing. You can thank the low-fat diet craze for that one.

So what did food companies do? They separated egg whites from the yolks. There's a problem with that, though. Most of the nutrients in eggs are found in the yolks. When you separate egg whites from the yolks, you are robbing yourself of many great key nutrients. It turns out that eggs contain all the vitamins the body needs except vitamin C.

Read that again: Whole eggs contain all the vitamins the body needs except vitamin C.

I can hear you saying, "But I don't like eggs." But do you like wellness, vitality, and healthy skin? You owe it to yourself to develop your palate to appreciate more of what allows you to be your very best. If it's a texture thing, that could mean cooking your eggs over hard versus over easy. If it's a flavor thing, that could mean preparing egg salad with flavorful herbs and spices rather than eating simple boiled eggs.

The egg yolk itself contains high amounts of vitamins A, D, E, K, B1, B3, B5, B6, B7, B9, and B12. Egg whites contain significant amounts of B1, B2, B3, B5, B6, B8, B9, and B12.

So if cooked beef liver is not your jam, get ready to enjoy some hard-boiled eggs. Eggs are a valuable source of choline, second only to beef liver. Choline is a nutrient that's responsible for memory, function, cognition, improved metabolism, healthy liver function, cell repair, mood, and DNA synthesis. When it comes to foggy memory and loss of cognition, choline plays a vital role in both. While the body makes choline in the liver, the amount is not enough to supply all you need. That is definitely something you want to think about to keep your brain active and healthy as you age.

Eggs also contain trace minerals such as selenium, calcium, copper, phosphorus, iron, and zinc. A deficiency in many of these same minerals is indicated in depression, fatigue, and chronic illnesses.

To get the most nutrients when eating eggs, buy eggs from egg-laying hens that are pasture-raised and free to roam and forage. Avoid eggs from battery-caged hens that eat a conventional diet. When you're enjoying eggs from pasture-raised hens, you'll notice that the yolks are dark yellow to orange in color versus light or pale yellow.

The bottom line? Boxed egg whites may seem healthy and convenient, but along with the missing yolk, you're also missing vitamins and nutrients. In addition, while conventional eggs may be more affordable, you're not getting a nutritional bang for your buck. Ultimately, when you consider the cost of illness and disease, it's more expensive to eat nutrient-poor foods since it leads to a sicklier, shorter life.

Many chronic diseases, illnesses, and conditions manifest not because of genetics or even aging but because of lifestyle choices, uncontrolled inflammation, and depletion of vitamins and micronutrients. We'll talk more about that in later chapters. Basically, you'll be doing yourself a lot of good simply by having two eggs a day.

Are You Allergic to Eggs?

While eating eggs is incredibly nutritious, delicious, and cost-effective, none of this actually matters if you're allergic to eggs. So if you're allergic and want to get more choline into your diet, try adding these choline-rich foods:

Grass-fed beef
Beef liver
Brussels sprouts
Seafood
Shiitake mushrooms
Chicken
Turkey
Almonds

DR. LISA'S NOTES

» When consuming foods with fats (as you should), consider the type of fat, the source, and how it was grown, raised, or prepared.
» It's beneficial to add a healthy fat such as olive oil or avocado oil to dark leafy greens before consuming for better absorption of nutrients.
» Fatty wild fish such as salmon are a great source of disease-fighting nutrients and omega-3 fats, but they are often mislabeled and adulterated. Do your research, and source them from reliable suppliers to make sure you're getting the real thing.
» Eat the whole egg!

WELLNESS PRESCRIPTION

» Invest in a good fish oil supplement. Get one that is wild-sourced, non-GMO, and free of artificial flavors and colors. Add it to your regimen today.

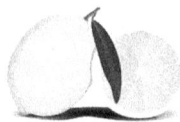

Chapter 13

ORGANIC FOOD PHARMACY

*Paying for your health on the front end
versus the back end is less expensive.*

During my coursework for my undergraduate science degree, I had to take a class in organic chemistry. I enjoyed adjusting the atom manipulatives and creating various types of chemical bonds. But organic chemistry was not my favorite class. One of the things the professor worked hard to drive home was that "organic" is anything with a carbon backbone.

He made it a point to tell us that chemically, all this talk about organic food was nonsense because all food is organic due to the presence of a carbon backbone. This was a nerdy joke of sorts, but the concept planted its way into my subconscious nevertheless.

It would take years before I understood firsthand the negative effects of chemical farming and why it's best to not have these harmful chemicals in our food. Oddly, organic farming was quite the norm throughout the 1920s before "conventionally grown" produce became the new normal.

As the population grew, technology advanced, food production increased, and the nutrition in that food continued to decline. Sure, you can grow tomatoes as big as your head when you use pesticides and synthetic fertilizers, but are the tomatoes equally as nutritious and just as tasty? And can you be certain there are zero negative health ramifications when choosing chemicals over nature?

Absolutely not.

THE DIRTY DOZEN AND CLEAN 15

When nourishing to flourish, it's important to eat the cleanest and freshest produce possible. Ideally, it should *all* be organic produce. If you can't afford to go all organic in the beginning, stick to avoiding the Dirty Dozen while focusing on eating the Clean 15.

The Dirty Dozen is a list of conventional fruits and vegetables that are almost always certain to have the most pesticide residue. Even if you're trying to save money at the grocery store, it's worth spending a bit more to purchase these products organically. On the latter, the Clean 15 are a list of conventional produce with the lowest pesticide residue.

Better ideas for saving money, than skipping organic produce, at the grocery store are to never go grocery shopping when you are hungry, shop in season, and avoid buying prepackaged foods. You'll get more nutrition out of your food that way too.

The list of Dirty Dozen foods is updated every year. On that list, you'll often find the usual suspects such as apples, strawberries, peaches, kale, grapes, bell peppers, tomatoes, cherries, grapes, nectarines, and pears. The top three on the Dirty Dozen list are apples, strawberries, and grapes.

When you're shopping organic, you're paying for your health on the front end (at the grocery store) by paying a bit more for organic produce. The alternative approach is saving more at the grocery store but paying more for your health at the back end. That happens with the money and time spent at the pharmacy, hospitals, avoidable surgeries, and countless doctors' visits. At the end of the day, it's really about perspective.

Ultimately, paying on the back end costs more money and time. So buy organic produce at the grocery store, and if you're really trying to save money, be sure to buy in season.

The More You Know, the More You Glow!

The Dirty Dozen are produce with the highest pesticide residue. If you want to enjoy these fruits and vegetables, buy them all organic, all the time. While chemically they all do have a carbon backbone, this is not about organic chemistry. This is about your health and well-being. Eventually, your goals should be to eat as close to 100 percent organic as possible.

The lists of the Dirty Dozen and the Clean 15 may change slightly from year to year, but generally, there are fruits and vegetables you can expect on the list. Remember, anything on the Dirty Dozen list should always be purchased organically due to the presence of pesticide and chemical residues. The items on the Clean 15 list are naturally low in pesticides; however, strive to purchase 100 percent organic when possible.

The Dirty Dozen

Strawberries
Spinach
Kale
Nectarines
Apples
Grapes
Peaches
Cherries
Pears
Tomatoes

Clean 15

Avocados
Sweet corn (not recommended on the Be FINE plan)
Pineapples
Cabbage
Onions
Sweet peas
Papayas
Asparagus
Eggplant
Honeydews
Kiwis
Cantaloupe
Cauliflower
Broccoli

ADDITIVES

Besides toxic chemicals and pesticides, there are other things to consider when grocery shopping. Certain food additives are harmful, cause inflammation, and lead to dire consequences to health.

As a matter of fact, it may surprise you to learn that some food additives are banned or have restricted use in Europe and other countries, but are still allowed in America.

You may ask, "Why would these food additives be banned in other countries?" Well, there's evidence that they cause harm to human health. These additives have been shown to contribute to hyperactivity in kids, inflammation, heart disease, diabetes, cancer, weight gain, and many more.

Here's a look at some food additives you should be on the lookout for and avoid. Yellow #5, yellow #6, red #40, partially hydrogenated oils (trans fats), BHA, BHT, potassium bromate, high fructose corn syrup, aspartame, monosodium glutamate, and brominated vegetable oil (BVO).

THE STANDARD AMERICAN DIET (SAD)

There's a reason that the "standard American diet" forms the acronym SAD. This modern diet is full of chemicals and is a sad excuse for nutrients, vitality, and health. Does it surprise you that as of this writing, the United States ranks number 27 when it comes to healthcare? That's not healthcare—it's "sickcare." Its great at emergency medicine and suppressing symptoms but not so great at wellness and preventative care.

If your goal is to be as healthy as possible, don't become a long-term customer of the healthcare system. To do so, you have to avoid the SAD diet. You must also be willing to educate yourself outside the doors of your doctor's office, pharma-funded research, and digital programming.

The question is, "Are you willing to do the work necessary to get there?"

DR. LISA'S NOTES

» The Dirty Dozen is a group of conventional fruits and vegetables with the highest pesticide residue.
» The Clean 15 is a group of conventional fruits and vegetables with the lowest pesticide residue.
» When grocery shopping, the goal should always be to source organic.

WELLNESS PRESCRIPTION

» For your next trip to the grocery store, ensure that at least 50 percent of your produce is organic. The ultimate goal is 100 percent organic within six months.

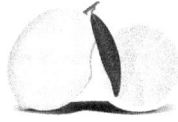

Chapter 14

FOOD BREAKS

*If you really want to get healthier, be willing
to trade your excuses for solutionss.*

I was extremely nauseous. One bite, and I knew I'd be hurling face-first over a toilet. Seventeen at that time, I don't remember what I had eaten. All I knew was that I didn't want to eat anything else after that. A well-intended family friend insisted that I have some chicken soup to help me feel better. Begrudgingly, I took a few small spoonfuls. Not long after the spoonfuls were in my mouth, I threw up all over the dining room floor. I didn't need food at that moment, and my body instinctively knew it. What I needed was a *food break*.

Truthfully, there are times when your body just doesn't need food.

You may be nauseous. You may be fasting. You may be ill. You may be tired. You may just be healing. No matter what you've heard, believe it or not, there are times in life when your body just doesn't need any food. In fact, voluntarily narrowing your eating window to between eight and twelve hours is actually a good thing.

Some people refer to this method of eating as *intermittent fasting* or *time-restricted eating*, although they are slightly different things.

While intermittent fasting includes some level of calorie restriction, time-restricted eating focuses specifically on narrowing the available eating window.

BENEFITS OF INTERMITTENT FASTING

The constant availability of food whenever and however we want it has led to an uptick in obesity, insulin resistance, hypertension, and more. I'm not talking about food scarcity. I'm talking about limiting food intake when you just don't need to eat.

Many ancient civilizations and religious subsets practiced and continue to practice some degree of fasting. They include Judaism, Buddhism, Hinduism, Islam, Christianity, and more. Jesus fasted in the wilderness and even gave instructions at the Sermon on the Mount on how to fast. When humans lived in the Paleolithic period, there were no all-you-can-eat buffets, 24-hour grocery stores, or the convenience of food delivery services. You either had food or you didn't.

Cyclically, there were periods of food availability and periods of famine. In more modern times, wars presented another challenge that affected food availability. Even so, it is apparent that fasting has been important throughout many civilizations. Is it simply coincidental that the appetite diminishes during certain times and types of illness? The Greek physician Hippocrates recommended food abstinence in times of certain illness and is attributed to saying, "To eat when you're sick is to feed your illness."

There are many benefits of fasting that are well-documented. To demonstrate this, here are some fast facts.

FAST FASTING FACTS

- Promotes better sleep
- Activates weight loss
- Clearer skin
- Decreases biological age (age based on cellular or DNA aging)
- Detoxification
- Decreased wrinkles
- Improves mental acuity
- Aids in wound healing

- Amplifies appetite regulation
- Metabolic flexibility
- Sharpens insulin sensitivity
- Increases energy
- Reduces stress
- Has an anti-cancer effect
- Autophagy (explained further below)
- Increases lifespan

You might be wondering, "How does the body produce energy in a state of food abstinence?" The lack of sugar coming into the body during fasting forces the body to burn other things for energy. The liver is a key component in converting non-carbohydrate materials such as amino acids and fats into glucose energy. The body can also break down body fat to make ketones, which act as an alternate source of energy.

AUTOPHAGY

In Greek, the word *autophagy* means "eat self" or "eating one's self." It's actually quite normal; autophagy is a natural phenomenon that occurs when specific cells in the body, called lysosomes, repair and break down damaged cells and proteins. That occurs in the absence of external food for fuel. While autophagy occurs in the body naturally, there are things you can do to amp it up even more.

You can think of this process like pruning a tree. Pruning leads to a healthier and stronger plant. In the case of humans, some of the benefits of autophagy include decreased cancer risk, mental clarity, and the elimination of toxins, which in turn leads to decreased disease risk.

There are also hormonal benefits to autophagy, including reduced insulin production, increased human growth hormone factor (HGF), and increased glucagon.

Glucagon is a hormone that cues the breakdown of glycogen into glucose in the body. Glycogen is just energy in the form of glucose.

Now back to glucagon. This is beneficial during periods of fasting since it helps to raise low blood sugar levels. These kinds of hormonal changes are the keys to aging well because they lead to controlled blood sugar, muscle growth, better sleep, radiant skin, improved energy, weight control, and much better health overall.

While autophagy can also be induced through things such as exercise and nutrition, one of the most documented and effective ways to induce autophagy is through intermittent fasting. Experts have differing opinions about exactly when autophagy is triggered during fasting. Some state that you need a minimum of twenty-four hours removed from food before autophagy is induced, while others say that a sixteen-hour food break followed by an eight-hour feeding window is enough to get the benefits. This is referred to as a 16:8 fast.

No matter which method you use, if you have preexisting conditions or are on prescription medication, before starting any fasting program, be sure to get guidance from a medical professional who is well-versed in this area. This is especially important if you want to press beyond 16 hours.

Feel free to adapt intermittent fasting to suit your lifestyle and activity. Some variations are weekdays on and weekends off, alternate day fasting, or reserving this way of fasting based on activity level and other lifestyle activities.

We'll talk more about fasting in the pages ahead.

NAD+

Any fine book about optimal wellness should at least include a section devoted to nicotinamide adenine dinucleotide (NAD or NAD+). And since this is not just any "fine" book but the FINE book, I'm here to deliver.

Let's make this as simple as possible.

Ready?

Let's go!

NAD+ is a coenzyme found in every cell of the body. It's responsible for DNA repair and energy production. It's also known as the key to healthy aging. As you age, NAD+ levels drop naturally, increasing DNA damage, age-related diseases, and more visible signs of aging. Once age fifty rolls around, you're likely to have half the NAD+ levels you had when you were twenty. NAD+ is available in the form of pills and IV therapy.

While commercially available, the best NAD+ you can get is made naturally by your own body. Fasting is one of the most effective ways to boost NAD+ levels, and the benefits of those boosted levels are many.

- Reduced weight gain
- Radiant skin
- Decrease incidence of neurodegenerative disease
- Improved exercise performance
- Increased lifespan

Here's the bottom line. If I could give you a longevity pill that would cost you nothing and even end up saving you money, would you take it? Of course you would! The restoration of NAD+ is one the biggest benefits of fasting.

So what are you waiting for?

Better get on this . . . FAST.

KEYS TO A SUCCESSFUL INTERMITTENT FAST

Our bodies were built to take scheduled breaks from eating. Hence, fasting was built into human life by design. When you sleep every night, your body naturally fasts for a period of time. Normal adults need anywhere from seven to nine hours of sleep every night. That means for seven to nine hours, you don't eat. You're fasting while your body restores and renews during the sleep cycle.

Hence, the first meal of the day is called "breakfast," which is made up of two words: "break" and "fast"—literally break the fast. The goal of intermittent fasting is to lengthen that natural fasting window.

The idea of an intermittent fast means you only eat during a specified eating window. There are many ways to do intermittent fasting. You can tailor this approach to certain days of the week or certain hours of the day. If you're just starting out, you'll want to ease your way in, perhaps lengthening the window of food abstinence to ten hours at first and then twelve. That would mean twelve hours of fasting with a twelve-hour feeding window. If you're game, you can extend this food break window to sixteen hours. While autophagy is not initiated during a twelve-hour fasting window, there are benefits of refraining from food regardless.

During this restricted window of eating, it's important to stay hydrated with plenty of clean water and keep up with electrolytes (in the form of Himalayan or wild salts). You can also have sugarless, antioxidant-rich teas (e.g., green teas, white teas) since they will not break your fast.

This is not the time for coconut water since coconuts are actually fruits, and drinking coconut water during your restricted eating window will break the fast. Fancy electrolyte sports drinks are also not recommended due to their sugar content and presence of artificial colors and flavors.

The point of this is not about eating less (although naturally that will occur); it's about restricting the eating window to a smaller period of time.

NOT SO FAST: IMPORTANT ELECTROLYTES

The benefits of fasting sound wonderful, don't they? But before you decide to jump on the bandwagon, not so fast! When you limit food intake for twelve hours or more, you are not only getting substantially less food but your body is also missing out on key electrolytes.

Electrolytes are minerals in the body that carry an electric charge. Some of these minerals include sodium, magnesium, and potassium. Inside the body, these electrolytes are responsible for many key processes, including maintaining hydration, nerve function, muscle contraction, and heart regulation. We get most of our electrolytes from the foods we eat.

In addition, during periods of fasting, insulin levels decrease. That causes the body to release water and sodium through the kidneys. In an effort to maintain electrolyte balance, potassium, magnesium, and calcium are also released.

This loss of electrolytes can have serious consequences. Early warning signs that you're not getting enough electrolytes include sluggishness, grumpiness, muscle cramps, and headaches.

To avoid this, make sure you're taking electrolytes during your fast. The key is to use non-sugar electrolytes that won't break your fast. You can do that by taking electrolyte waters. Remember, sports drinks, fruit juices, artificially flavored waters, and even coconut water are not advised.

Sugar-free electrolyte mixes that won't break your fast are easy to buy, but you can also make your own at home.

Fast, Friendly Electrolyte Drink

8 oz plain or spring water (do not use flavored waters or tonic water)
2 tbsp lime or lemon juice
1 tbsp unpasteurized apple cider vinegar
1 tsp unrefined Himalayan salt

HOW TO BREAK AN INTERMITTENT FAST

The constant availability of food, coupled with a grazing mentality of steady consumption, turns off all the body's opportunities for detoxification, autophagy, and metabolic flexibility. These natural processes are some of the keys to aging healthfully, preventing disease, and enabling restoration.

Whatever time you break your intermittent fast, choose a balanced, high-protein meal using these *fast breakers* for a powerful start.

Fast Breakers

Boiled eggs
Wild caught fish
Quinoa
Raw nuts
Bone broth
Protein-rich green smoothies
Soups
Pasture-raised chicken
Non-GMO, organic, raw, or gently cooked fruits and vegetables
Grass-fed, grass-finished meat
Wild rice (this does not contain actual rice; don't get a wild rice blend or mix)

After you've broken the fast, other foods to consider during the specified feeding window are non-GMO and organic vegetables, wild-caught fish, pasture-raised meats, raw nuts, grain-free starches, grass-fed ghee, and fresh fruits.

While intermittent fasting is a powerful tool, it's not for everybody.

There continues to be a myriad of benefits associated with varied degrees of fasting. These include the reversal of diabetes, lowering high lipid levels, treatment and mitigation of cancer, weight loss, hormonal and thyroid imbalance, and other positive effects for those with chronic diseases.

Certain groups, like those taking insulin to lower their blood sugar, may suffer from unpredictable hypoglycemia, or low blood sugar. If this is you, I strongly urge you to work with your medical team, including a naturopath who is well-versed in working with patients in this category so you can be closely monitored.

Intermittent Fasting May Not Be Ideal If You:

- Are underweight
- Are under eighteen
- Are pregnant
- Are breastfeeding
- Have metabolic conditions such as type 1 diabetes
- Are on insulin or other blood-sugar-lowering medication
- Have a history of eating disorders

If you have any concerns or questions, consult your healthcare provider.

DR. LISA'S NOTES

» Fasting is a practice that has been around for thousands of years.
» Limiting food intake to specific shortened eating windows has a myriad of health benefits.

WELLNESS PRESCRIPTION

» Work on shortening your eating window this week. Have your first meal one hour later and your last meal one hour earlier. The goal is to find an intermittent fasting window that works for you.

INFLAMMATION AND IMMUNITY

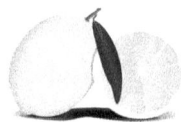

Chapter 15

INFLAMMATION

*Fake food is like fake people. Eventually the
toxicity will come out and really start to stink.*

We spent a lot of time in the previous chapters talking about food—what kind to eat, what nutrients you can get from it, where to buy it, and even why you sometimes need to take breaks from it. The reason so much of this book is spent on food is because fueling with the wrong types of foods continues to be a driving force for chronic inflammation. You'll recall that when your body activates your immune system in response to an attack, it sends out inflammatory cells. These cells attack bacteria or heal damaged tissue. But if your body sends out inflammatory cells when you're *not* sick or injured, you may develop chronic inflammation, which is damaging to your body.

If you reduce chronic inflammation, you also improve immunity, promote healthy aging, decrease disease, and increase longevity.

Is it just me, or does it seem like the definition of what and who is "healthy" keeps changing every day?

According to the media, what is considered healthy today is not necessarily healthy tomorrow. Just so you know, it takes an average of 17 years for scientific research to reach the clinical setting. What does that mean exactly? It means you can't solely depend on your physician or TV screen to tell you what to do for good health.

As a matter of fact, there's a huge conflict of interest when it comes to receiving unbiased information from these sources in order to attain better health.

That's why chasing current health fads is not the answer. It's much more effective to develop long-term wellness practices that lean on natural medicine as a first line of defense to wholeness and well-being.

I call this becoming "whealthy."

It's a way to take control of your health and wellness by strengthening your body's own natural immune function. Doing that suppresses unwanted inflammation and disease.

That's why you can't talk about inflammation without referencing immunity. They go together like almond butter and raw honey—I mean sunrise and sunsets—well, summer and sandals. Pretty much when you think of one, you have to consider the other.

Mainstream health is based on approaches from the "outside in," whereas wellness and being whealthy takes an "inside out" approach.

Once you understand that, you have the power. The only thing left is to take it and learn how to use it to your benefit. That's where inflammation and immunity come into play.

First, let's talk about inflammation and why it's important. There are lots of facets that affect inflammation. Many of them were discussed in the "F" part of FINE. They are mainly things like GMOs, pesticides, artificial colors and flavors, dairy, allergies, omega-6 fats, and grain, which can all cause inflammation.

This inflammation is not just limited to the gut. Devastatingly, it can find itself all over the body. But all inflammation is not created equal. In fact there are two types of inflammation: acute and chronic.

Acute inflammation has a sudden onset and is the body's appropriate response to injury. It's a temporary condition and part of the body's natural healing process.

On the contrary, chronic inflammation has no "off" button. Long-term, chronic inflammation can cause serious damage and is the basis of most diseases. Whether that inflammation is caused by stress, food, environment, illness, or injury, you have to get to the bottom of the triggers.

The good news is that most of those triggers can be controlled.

You may have heard that chronic inflammation is caused by things like "bad" genes, autoimmune disorders, toxins, bacteria, and chemical exposure—in other words, things you can't necessarily control. While some of that is true, what caused those genes to be activated? What triggered the autoimmune disorder, and is there a source behind the chronic inflammation?

The majority of times, you can do something about it.

Let's take food, for example. The reason that food is a source of both wellness and illness is because eating is one of the things you do multiple times a day, so there is a huge opportunity for impact. Let's say that you eat three meals and two snacks a day. That's five opportunities you have to either control inflammation or make things worse.

Imagine inflammation as a small fire in your body. You can either throw some kerosene on the dry brush, watch it flare up, and walk away; or you can extinguish the flames, smother the embers, and continuously saturate the area with water. These are two different courses of action with two different sets of results. And when it comes to inflammation, there are many fire enablers or forms of "kerosene" that you need to be aware of.

This is not about vilifying foods. It's about empowerment so you are not inadvertently led down the wrong path while being a slave to your taste buds.

Some of the top inflammatory foods include grains, dairy, artificial colors, genetically modified crops, processed foods, artificial dyes, grain-fed meat, and sugar.

Yes, we're back on sugar. In chapter 11, I talked about the prevalence of sugar, the many names for it, and how it directly correlates with metabolic disease, weight gain, unhealthy aging, and illness. Are you ready for another truth bomb?

Most people are unknowingly dining on foods that cause inflammation several times a day.

Combine those food choices with sedentary lifestyles, stress, inadequate sleep, food intolerances, and the toxic stew of chemicals that people eat, wear, and breathe, and what you have is a ticking time bomb ready to go off at any given moment. Fortunately, you have control over most of these things. The biggest variable, of course, is food.

As a reminder, sugar and seed oils are some of the biggest instigators of chronic inflammation.

The sneaky thing about chronic inflammation is that you won't know it's there until things start breaking down. That may or may not lead to a clinical diagnosis. Until then, you could be exposing yourself to triggers of inflammation over and over again and not even be aware of it. The human body is highly adaptive and sophisticated. Inflammatory responses start at a cellular level and can fester for years before they're detected.

Some conditions that result from chronic inflammation are auto-immune disorders such as Crohn's disease, type 1 diabetes, lupus, and rheumatoid arthritis. Besides autoimmune diseases, other conditions due to chronic inflammation include heart disease, cancer, and numerous degenerative disorders. To fight this, you must be aware of the common inflammatory triggers and avoid them as much as possible. Diet, of course, is one of the biggest inflammatory triggers and simultaneously the low-hanging fruit of how to get your life back.

Do you see how much what you eat matters? You literally can't ignore this aspect if you truly want to be FINE.

Since chronic inflammation is so sneaky, being proactive is paramount. You have to look for it first, or it may come looking for you. One of the ways to do that is by asking for a C-reactive protein (CRP) test during your next physical. This test measures chronic inflammation by detecting the CRP protein found in the blood. A slight drawback with this test is that you can't tell where the inflammation is coming from.

If you're concerned about heart inflammation, a more specific test to ask for is the high sensitivity C-reactive protein test, or hs-CRP test. Due to this test's increased sensitivity, it's used to determine future heart attack risk.

GOOD INFLAMMATION

There are different types of inflammation in the body. It may surprise you to learn that some inflammation is actually good. When you get injured or are fighting infection, the body promotes localized inflammation as a way to help the body heal. You're able to relate to this if you've ever gotten a cut or scrape. The body sends white blood cells to the area, resulting in temporary redness and swelling. This disappears as the wound heals naturally, and soon the area looks normal again.

However, continuous or chronic inflammation is not good.

DR. LISA'S NOTES

» Inflammation can be either acute or chronic.
» Acute inflammation is a healthy and necessary part of bodily function and healing.
» Chronic inflammation can indicate serious damage and a sign of disease.

WELLNESS PRESCRIPTION

» Let's get real! Name the main food that is a source of inflammation for you. Write the name here: _____.

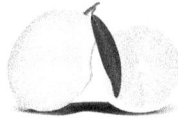

Chapter 16

INFLAMMAGING AND HEALTHSPAN

Don't deny or misrepresent the amount of years
God has blessed you with. If you do, the chances
are good he'll summon you to talk about it.

The topic of aging is not necessarily met with warmth and joy by everyone.

Recently, a woman celebrated her thirtieth birthday. After thanking everyone for their birthday wishes, she went on to complain about the fact that no one mentioned all the joint pain she would be having once she hit thirty. While it surprised me to hear her say that, what surprised me even more was the number of people who affirmed her with stories of their own.

Were her observations justified? Is joint pain over thirty a normal sign of aging, or is it a sign of *inflammaging*?

Inflammaging is rapid aging due to chronic inflammation.

While people are welcome to share their individual perspectives and experiences, it's important to note that healthy aging is not characterized by pain, bowel disturbances, memory loss, forgetfulness, decreased mobility, or chronic illness. These are signs and symptoms of inflammaging, which is often more prevalent and normalized in industrialized nations. It shows up in joints, brain, skin, intestines, and wherever else it wants to go.

It's important to note that inflammaging is not due to aging itself but to the dietary and lifestyle choices that precede it. As a result, inflammaging often leads to a mischaracterization of getting old.

Hence, while lifespan is important, your *healthspan* is even more crucial. You can live a long life and still be in chronic debilitating pain every day. Healthspan is a better indicator of health and vitality. Your age is what you make it. Be grateful for every year you've been given, and make those years count while steering clear of inflammation.

Don't deny or misrepresent the amount of years you think God has blessed you with. If you do, the chances are good he'll summon you to talk about it.

ANTI-INFLAMMATORY SUPER POWER

When it comes to decreasing inflammation, there are some heavy-hitting, anti-inflammatory powerhouses you should definitely add to your regimen. The choices are numerous, but I want to highlight a few of the A-listers. That doesn't mean that other foods don't have antioxidant, anti-inflammatory, and immune-boosting power. These are just my favorites.

The fabulous thing about using food as medicine is that you don't need a prescription to take advantage of it. In addition, *functional cooking* is a great way to reap the benefits of both anti-inflammatory and immune-building foods.

Functional cooking is a way of improving the nutrition and health benefits of foods without sacrificing flavor. Oftentimes, making just a few ingredient swaps can make a big impact on nutrition.

Here are some easy swaps you could try:

- Instead of white flour, use nut flours made from almonds or chickpeas.
- Substitute pureed vegetables for half of the ground beef in a recipe for added nutrition.
- Use wild rice in place of white rice.
- Use more herbs.
- Trade processed salt for wild-sourced, Celtic, or Himalayan salt.
- Instead of bread or flour tortillas, use lettuce or leafy greens to make wraps.

- Choose toasted nuts or raw nuts instead of croutons.
- Try spiralized or riced vegetables in place of pasta and rice.
- Instead of soy sauce, try liquid coconut aminos.
- If you're craving noodles, use zoodles (zucchini noodles) or spaghetti squash.
- Use unsweetened almond milk or coconut milk instead of traditional milk (macadamia milk is also a great alternative and has a creamy texture).
- For breakfast, try swapping your oatmeal for ground flaxseed or quinoa with unsweetened nut milk.
- Replace canola oil with coconut oil or olive oil when cooking.

When it comes to anti-inflammatory foods, there are some heavy hitters that stand out. From fruits to spices and herbs, let's go a little deeper so you can stock up on the right ingredients and have your food work for you and not against you.

Turmeric (Curcumin)

A yellow fragrant spice known for its vibrant color, turmeric has been touted as one of the most powerful antioxidants and anti-inflammatory agents in the world. As one of the main ingredients in curry powder, turmeric is a potent anti-inflammatory. The anti-inflammatory benefits in turmeric are due to curcuminoids. Curcumin, the active ingredient in turmeric, is associated with longevity, metabolism, glucose metabolism, and gut health.

As a Caribbean native, one of my favorite ways to enjoy turmeric is in a hearty bowl of curry chicken. Some other easy ways to enjoy turmeric is in a cup of warm, golden milk or adding the spice to your favorite soups and stews.

The benefits of curcumin have been demonstrated in chronic illnesses such as Alzheimer's, osteoarthritis, rheumatoid arthritis, cancer, skin ailments, and aging.

As much as curcumin is impressive, you have to eat a lot of turmeric to get the therapeutic amount you need. Hence, supplementation is key. Since curcumin is not readily absorbed by the body, it's necessary to make a few adjustments to enhance absorption. The addition of piperine in supplements, also known as black pepper extract, is one of those ways. Piperine increases the absorption of curcumin in the blood by 2,000 percent.

Another way to increase the bioavailability of curcumin is by taking it in liposomal form. Taking a liposomal form of curcumin allows for easier absorption by the body.

Fermented turmeric is yet another way to enhance curcumin absorption.

No matter which turmeric supplement you buy, be mindful of artificial colors that are sometimes added to increase the color and appeal of the product. While it's not a must, a curcumin supplement that contains ginger can work synergistically to improve anti-inflammatory effects.

Ginger

Another very powerful anti-inflammatory food is ginger. Ginger is such a powerhouse that you're doing yourself a disservice if you don't have some in your kitchen. Also known as a rhizome, ginger has been used for at least 2,500 years. It's full of anti-inflammatory power. From digestive upset, nausea, pain relief, and even diabetes, the list of health benefits are long. Some of my personal favorite ways to use ginger are freshly grated in hot tea and added to stews, juices, and smoothies.

But however you decide to use ginger, you can't go wrong. Using some ginger is better than using no ginger at all.

Berries

Oh sookie, sookie now! Here comes my jam—no pun intended. Berries are known for their antioxidant power and prevention of free radicals that promote disease and premature aging. While most people think of blueberries only for their anti-inflammatory benefits, there are some other juicy gems you need to know about. Some have funny and hard-to-pronounce names, but I promise that you'll still want these as part of your wellness arsenal.

Acaí berry

Native to the Amazon rainforest, acai berries are one of nature's true superfoods. Since acai berries have such a short shelf life, it's likely that you won't be able to get fresh acai berries outside of where they are grown. Look for pureed acai berries in the freezer section of your grocery store or as a powder or juice. One of my favorite ways to enjoy acai berries is in deliciously prepared acai bowls.

Amla

Also known as Indian gooseberry, amla is a powerful antioxidant, anti-in-flammatory, and source of vitamin C with numerous medicinal properties. In Ayurvedic medicine, amla is praised for its wound-healing and cardi-oprotective, neuroprotective, and gastroprotective properties.

But this is just the beginning. In addition, this medicinal plant has potent properties used in the prevention and treatment of cancer.

If you're considering adding this to your regimen, make sure to get one that is third-party tested. One of my favorite ways to take amla is adding it to smoothies. When used as a powder, less than a teaspoon is all you need.

Goji Berry

Goji berries are native to Asia and contain high levels of both antioxidants and nutrients. As a result, this superfood is great for eye health, helps to protect the liver and is beneficial in reducing blood sugar. You will most likely find these berries sun-dried or freeze dried at the grocery store. Goji berries are red and have a sweet and sour flavor. Snack on goji berries by themselves, or add them to homemade trail mix or grain-free granola.

Elderberry

While there are several types of elderberry, two common types—the European elderberry (*Sambucus nigra*) and the American elderberry (*Sambucus canadensis*)—are the ones you want. Specifically, the use of black elderberries have shown a reduction in duration and severity of the common cold and influenza. To get the most benefits from elderberries, get them in syrups, tinctures, capsules, and even gummies as an adjuvant to boost the immune system.

Cinnamon

Cinnamon is an incredibly powerful spice that is a sledgehammer to inflammation, an ally in decreasing chronic illness, and an asset to immunity. There are hundreds of kinds of cinnamon. But before we get into the nitty gritty, I want to bust your bubble . . . I mean, educate you for a second. Do you know that most of the cinnamon labeled and sold in grocery stores is not considered true cinnamon?

I know it's crazy, but please bear with me. True cinnamon comes from a tree native to Sri Lanka and Madagascar. It's called Ceylon Cinnamomum (*Cinnamomum zeylanicum*, or True Cinnamon).

Another plant, cassia (*Cinnamomum cassia*), is native to China, Vietnam, Indonesia, and India, and is more readily available. It's the most common form sold in the United States. While these spices can be used interchangeably, inherently they are not the same. Even Saigon cinnamon is a variety of cassia and is not true cinnamon.

There isn't one variety that is bad, but it's important to note that when you read about the benefits and health studies associated with cinnamon, you know which type of cinnamon is being referenced. Many of the more notable studies are associated with Ceylon cinnamon.

Cassia is more readily available, less expensive, and has a stronger flavor. Ceylon is lighter, milder in flavor, and more expensive. While this is the case, Ceylon cinnamon has significant anti-inflammatory effects, has been shown to be beneficial in diabetes, reducing LDL (low-density lipoprotein), raising HDL (high-density lipoprotein), reducing blood pressure, and much more. This is not to say that there are no health benefits associated with the other species of cinnamon. But when it comes to documented medicinal value, true cinnamon is more evidence-based. For example, when four commercially available types of cinnamon were compared for their anti-hyperglycemic value, Ceylon cinnamon came out on top.

Some healthy ideas for using more cinnamon in your meals include sprinkling it in tea, putting it on top of warm cereal, adding it to smoothies, and using it as a garnish on baked sweet potatoes.

Garlic

Love it or hate it, garlic (*allium sativum*) is here to stay. The benefits of garlic are well documented and have been used for thousands of years throughout civilizations. These anti-inflammatory effects are well touted in showing benefits in cancer prevention, reducing cholesterol levels, decreasing dementia, and helping fight infection. Whether you're enjoying it crushed, sliced, or whole, be sure to add some garlic to your next meal.

By the way, do yourself a favor. In the supermarket, walk past the bottle of pre-peeled, pre-crushed garlic. You have no idea how long it has been sitting there! Also, avoid buying garlic that is missing the roots.

This is why. It may surprise you to learn that China is one of the biggest importers of garlic sold in the US. Domesticated garlic has roots and imported garlic doesn't. This "rootless" garlic is bleached with a chemical that stops sprouting and then is often disinfected with methyl bromide, a known toxin that causes central nervous system and respiratory damage.

Basil

Praised for its antioxidant and anti-inflammatory benefits, basil is the herb you can't get enough of. As a matter of fact, I'm actually sipping on a cup of basil tea as I write this. There are more than sixty varieties of basil, and the health benefits spread far and wide. Holy basil (also known as tulsi), for example, has great medicinal value and has been used in Ayurvedic medicine. You can thank the essential oils in basil—eugenol, linalool, and citronellol—for the potent anti-inflammatory effects. You may also enjoy using some basil essential oil in a diffuser. A few drops go a long way, and it's so good!

Cayenne Pepper

Feeling hot, hot, hot! Whew! Thank goodness that cayenne and other hot peppers such as chili peppers have more to give than a burning sensation in the mouth. Capsaicin, the compound that gives cayenne pepper its kick, is responsible for the anti-inflammatory effects. These peppers help with everything from congestion, pain (from arthritis), metabolism, digestion, and more. The benefits of capsaicin are so well documented that you can even purchase capsaicin cream and patches to help with pain. So the next time you cook, add a couple shakes or slivers into the pot. You'll be healthier for it.

DR. LISA'S NOTES

» Inflammaging is a sign of unhealthy aging due to chronic inflammation.
» Lifespan and healthspan are not the same thing.
» Make simple food swaps and additions to meals for increased anti-inflammatory superpower.

WELLNESS PRESCRIPTION

» Look at the food items under "Anti-Inflammatory Super Power," and select three ingredients to add to your meal this week. (Hint: It can be something as simple as sprinkling some cayenne pepper on a salad.)

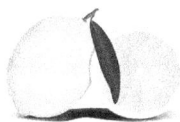

Chapter 17

YOU'RE SUCH A TEAS

The best teas don't come in a bag.

We can't talk about inflammation and immunity without talking about tea. True tea comes from one plant—the tea plant—scientifically known as *Camellia sinensis*. Different levels of oxidation and fermentation of this one plant provide different varieties of tea such as white tea, green tea, black tea, and oolong tea.

White tea is the least processed of the bunch and contains the most antioxidants, while black tea is the most processed and oxidized.

Tea is a phenomenal tool in the battle against inflammation, unwanted disease, unhealthy aging, and cancer. Not only is drinking hot tea relaxing, but compounds in tea called polyphenols and catechins are potent and work to give the body exactly what it needs.

These polyphenols act as antioxidants that prevent free radicals from causing damage to the body. Antioxidants are one of the major work-horses of health and wellness.

These tea polyphenols consist mostly of catechins. The most powerful of these is epigallocatechin gallate (EGCG).

Free radicals are the unstable, highly reactive compounds in the body that form during normal metabolic processes or are introduced from the environment. These free radicals have been linked to atherosclerosis, inflammaging, cancer, and other diseases. An increased intake of anti-oxidants minimizes the risk of health problems posed by free radicals.

In addition to the above benefits, green tea extract has fat-burning properties that promote weight loss. That is especially beneficial when combined with increased physical activity and a healthy diet.

So drop the iced tea, sweet tea, and powdery iced tea mixes. You'll get many more benefits by swapping those quick teas for slow teas.

TEA BUYING AND PREPARATION TIPS

Even though tea bags are an option when buying tea, opt for loose teas whenever possible. That is because tea bags are often made with "tea dust," which are lower quality small particles of tea that are bagged from scraps and sold. Studies have shown that the antioxidant levels of tea bags aren't up to par with loose, whole leaf tea. That doesn't mean you can never buy tea bags. It just means you have to be smart about the bagged tea you are buying. You can still get a lot of antioxidants from some premium bagged tea varieties. You just have to know what to get.

When buying tea bags, avoid flat tea bags whenever possible. If the tea bag is triangular or three-dimensional in shape, that's a good sign. Also make sure it's packaged in unbleached bags to avoid chemical residue and toxin exposure.

If you're looking for the convenience of tea bags, you can buy loose tea leaves and bag them individually yourself. Again, make sure you're using unbleached tea bags. The use of tea ball strainers also allows users to steep a cup of their favorite brew while keeping tea leaves out of the way.

When it's time to make a cup of your favorite brew, remember that every tea has its own "temperament." There is both an ideal temperature and time required for steeping. Both are equally important, so pay close attention to what tea you have and how it likes to be treated. You can easily find this information on the package of your loose tea or tea bags.

Bringing water to a rolling boil, dropping in a tea bag in that water, and walking away for 20 minutes while you catch up on your favorite show is not called "making tea." It's called "burning the tea," and it tastes terrible. Respect the tea, treat the tea kindly, and the tea will respect you.

The best way to determine how long to steep a desired cup of tea is by checking the package it comes in. Here's a tea steeping guide you can use to get started.

Tea-Making Chart

Tea Type and How Long to Steep
　Black, 3–5 minutes
　Green, 2–3 minutes
　Oolong, 2–3 minutes
　White, 1–3 minutes

HERBAL TEAS

As far back as I can remember, herbal teas have been a staple in my life. While true tea comes from the *Camellia sinensis*, herbal teas are made from a variety of other plants and may include their roots, shoots, barks, and leaves. Herbal teas are also called tisanes or herbal infusions. Unlike true tea, herbal teas contain no natural caffeine unless they are combined with true tea.

Herbal teas are not only comforting but also soothing and healing. As a matter of fact, West Indians rely on tea so much that they often joke that there is nothing that a cup of tea can't cure. Menstrual cramps, headaches, sore throat, nausea, insomnia, body aches, or whatever—if you have it, there is a cup of tea best suited for it.

Unlike true teas, herbal teas need to be steeped a bit more to get the good stuff out. You'll want to allow a steep time of at least ten minutes. Other than that, your tea selection is only limited by your imagination and curiosity.

Here are some herbal tea selections you can try to get started.

Chamomile Tea

Chamomile tea calms your nerves, soothes, and encourages sleep. It also helps soothe muscle spasms experienced in menstrual cramps. The best chamomile tea is made from the flowers of the plant, not the leaves.

Basil Tea

Fresh basil leaves make a fragrant tea that can be enjoyed by itself or in combination with any herbal or true tea. Basil tea boasts many of the same anti-inflammatory benefits you come to expect from other powerful herbs and plants.

Garlic Tea

Fresh cloves of garlic boiled in water make a simple yet powerful tea chocked full of benefits. Garlic has anti-microbial, anti-inflammatory, and immune-boosting benefits. Garlic tea is a powerful aid for coughs, colds, and congestion.

Lemongrass Tea

I have fond memories of starting my mornings as a child and young adult drinking a cup of fresh lemongrass tea. It was never bagged and likely picked from someone's yard or garden that morning. Often, the tasty brew wasn't just lemongrass—it included other fresh herbs such as rosemary, thyme, and basil. No matter how you enjoy it, there's nothing like a cup of fresh lemongrass tea to get the day going.

Drinking lemongrass tea has been shown to relieve bloating, boost oral health, lower cholesterol, and reduce anxiety. And of course, there are anti-inflammatory effects.

I'll admit that when it comes to tea, I was spoiled by my island childhood and fresh herbal teas. To this day, seeing bagged, dried lemongrass tea at the store makes me want to run in the other direction. But you do the best you can!

Peppermint Tea

A cup of peppermint tea is quite invigorating. The leaves have anti-inflammatory and antimicrobial benefits. Drinking peppermint tea helps soothe the stomach and, when taken after a meal, can act as a digestive aid.

Red Raspberry Tea

If you menstruate, red raspberry tea is definitely a tea to have on hand since it eases uterine cramps. Like the other teas on this list, red raspberry tea has antioxidants as well as anti-inflammatory benefits.

Orange Peel Tea

You know the practice of tossing orange peels in the trash after feasting on the juicy fleshy fruit?

One word . . .

Don't!

As a matter of fact, I don't think I've ever seen my mom throw an orange peel in the trash. The sweet-smelling peels can be hung and dried to make aromatic tea. Orange peel tea contains vitamin C, a powerful antioxidant. The tea also has potent immunity-raising benefits and may even play a role in diabetes management.

Ginger Tea

Ginger is one of those spices you always want to have on hand. Not only is it a delicious addition to smoothies, soups, and stir-fries, but this root makes a potent tea either by itself or in combination with other teas.

One of ginger tea's claims to fame includes minimizing digestive upset such as nausea, queasy stomach, and diarrhea. It can reduce pain and aid in reducing blood pressure. Ginger also has cancer-fighting properties.

THE DECAF DILEMMA

If you drink tea, you probably drink tea for one of two reasons.

Reason number one is that obviously you enjoy it!

Reason number two is that you've heard about the immune-boosting, cancer-fighting benefits of tea.

Avid tea drinkers enjoy tea for both of these reasons. No matter what your reasons are for drinking tea, you should know that cancer despises tea. The natural polyphenols found in true tea are a cancer nemesis.

Now here comes the dilemma. You may want to enjoy those benefits without the caffeine. For that reason, some people turn to decaffeinated tea as an option.

If that's you, here are some things you should consider. While decaffeinated tea contains less caffeine than traditional tea, there's still *some* caffeine. In addition, the methods used to remove caffeine from tea are by no means holistic. Chemicals such as methylene chloride and ethyl acetate are often used to remove caffeine. In addition, some polyphenols and antioxidants are removed from tea during the decaffeination process. That means you get less caffeine but more chemicals and less health benefits per cup.

If you still have concerns about the caffeine in tea, feel encouraged that the average cup of tea contains less caffeine than a cup of coffee. In addition, herbal infusions (herbal tea) such as Tulsi basil and chamomile teas are naturally caffeine free!

DR. LISA'S NOTES

» There are two types of tea: true teas and herbal teas.
» Tea acts as a cancer preventer, immune booster, weight reducer, antioxidant producer, inflammation fighter, and vitality enhancer.
» True tea should be purchased as loose tea or in non-flat, unbleached bags whenever possible.

WELLNESS PRESCRIPTION

» Don't be a "teas"! Include at least one true tea or one herbal tea as part of your daily regimen. Drink two cups per day.

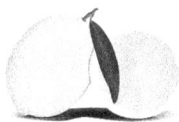

Chapter 18

IT'S TIME FOR A GUT CHECK

Some people won't be satisfied until they've done everything they can to disrupt your good gut flora.

You cannot have a thorough conversation about immunity without talking about the microbiome. The microbiome consists of about 39 trillion microbes, including bacteria, fungi, and viruses that live in and on the body including the feet, gastrointestinal tract, vagina, armpits, scalp, mouth, and all over the skin.

Many of these microbes live in the gut—the long tube from the mouth to the anus, officially known as the gastrointestinal tract (GI). Your mood, skin health, changes in weight, autoimmune conditions, and, of course, immunity are all impacted by gut health. It's not the gut by itself but the gut and the microbes that live there and in other parts of the body that run the show.

There are good gut flora and bad gut flora.

It's your job to make sure these microbes are in harmonious balance and happy. That goes beyond tossing in a few probiotics and thinking they will solve the problem. Eating crap all day, accompanied by crap with a side of more crap, rolled and dusted in premium crap, is like a sucker punch to the gut at every single meal. You wouldn't do that to your worst enemy.

But what you can't see won't hurt, right?

WRONG!

Since up to 80 percent of your immunity is in your gut, what's on the end of your fork really matters.

Here's why. As important as the gut is to overall wellness and immunity, it may surprise you to learn that the epithelial cells—the cells that cover the inside and outside of the surfaces of your body—that line the gut are only one cell layer thick.

These epithelial cells are super important since they facilitate the digestion of food and absorption of nutrients, and aid in protecting the body from pathogens that can cause illness and disease. Any compromise to this single cell layer can present a big problem.

Holes and perforations in the gut (known as leaky gut) can cause microscopic invaders such as partially digested food, mold, and toxins to have direct access to the bloodstream. These invaders can also increase the space between gap junctions, the tight spaces between epithelial cells. Gap junctions are the gatekeepers that control what moves in and out of the gut.

Certain foods such as gluten and dairy are notorious for causing these gaps to open up.

GMOs are also notorious for having devastating effects on the gut lining. They also are brimming with glyphosate, one of the most used pesticides in the world. Eighty-eight percent of wheat flour, 80 percent of pasta, 75 percent of oats, and mostly all wheat and cereal brands are contaminated with glyphosate.

Any changes in intestinal permeability can cause the immune system to make antibodies to poorly digested food and normal microflora. These leaks can cause chronic illness, autoimmune diseases, allergies, and a compromised immune system.

Besides GMOs and glyphosate, other causes of leaky gut include food additives, environmental pollutants, processed foods, and excessive drinking. Drugs and pharmaceutical treatments such as those found in birth control, aspirin, ibuprofen, steroids, and chemotherapy have also been implicated in creating prime conditions for leaky gut.

FOODS THAT DECREASE IMMUNITY AND ARE BAD FOR THE GUT

Sugar

If you want to improve your immunity, you have to limit sugar.

GMOs

GMOs, or genetically modified crops, contain glyphosate, which can have a devastating effect on overall health. Some of the most genetically modified crops are corn, cotton, soybeans, sugar, and canola.

In addition, it's a common practice to spray crops such as wheat and oats with glyphosate just prior to harvest for more consistent yield. This practice, of course, is harmful to humans.

Seed Oils and Foods High in Omega-6

As mentioned in Chapter 12, the ratio of omega-3 fats ingested should be higher than omega-6 fats. High levels of omega-6 oils are known catalysts for agitating the immune system. That alone is reason enough to seek out 100 percent grass-fed and pasture-raised meat and poultry. Studies show that 100 percent grass-fed beef and pasture-raised products have high amounts of omega-3. These fats are beneficial in decreasing inflammation and lowering the chances of cardiovascular disease, stroke, and cancer.

When it comes to poultry and eggs, pasture-raised animal products also have higher amounts of omega-3 fats compared to conventionally raised. Just crack open a conventional egg and compare it side by side with a pasture-raised egg, and you'll see the sunshine yellow-orange difference. Pasture-raised eggs taste better too!

Processed Foods

The general rule of thumb is that if your great-grandmother would not recognize it as food, you want to avoid it. Processed foods also have unwanted additives, colors, flavors, and preservatives.

Refined Carbohydrates

Refined carbohydrates are quickly broken down into sugar and cause insulin spikes, which are associated with chronic disease and illness. These carbohydrates also provide food for bad bacteria in the gut, causing their overgrowth and an imbalance of good and bad bacteria.

KEY TO GOOD GUT HEALTH

In addition to avoiding trigger foods, there are some other habits for good gut health that help foster a strong immune system and better overall wellness. When it comes to gut health, most people are eager to talk about *probiotics* but neglect the importance of *prebiotics* and the role they play in the maintenance of healthy gut flora. Prebiotics are plant fibers that feed the good bacteria in the gut, whereas probiotics are bacteria and yeast that are added to the diet to support a healthy gut.

Prebiotics: Gut-Friendly Foods to Feed Your Bugs

As I've already mentioned, humans are pretty "buggy." In you and on you are trillions of microscopic bugs, including bacteria, viruses, and fungi. It's pretty much a cohabitation situation. Just like a good roommate, you have to do right by your bugs if you want your bugs to do right by you.

That all starts with food.

Be sure to add prebiotic foods to your gut-friendly menu. Cruciferous vegetables such as cabbage, Romanesco, Brussels sprouts, broccoli sprouts, kale, and cabbage are mainstays and have potent anticancer benefits. Garlic, apples, turmeric, onions, and leeks are gut-friendly and easy additions to support a healthy gut.

So that covers feeding the healthy bacteria that are already there, but if you want to add more good bacteria to the mix, you're going to have to add probiotics.

Probiotics: Good Bacteria

The addition of probiotics to your wellness strategy is a worthy consideration for good health. Probiotics are more than about immune boosting; they support good gut health that is necessary for healthy skin, improved mood, and good bowel habits. They even help with seasonal allergies.

If you're having an issue tolerating high-fiber foods, the addition of probiotic-containing foods such as traditionally fermented sauerkraut to your diet can help to improve the breakdown and digestion of those foods. Of course, you can take a probiotic supplement to get some of those good bugs, but there is so much you can do with food. So let's start there.

Be FINE Probiotic Foods:

Kombucha
Kimchi
Pickles (make sure they're the old-school fermented pickles)
Sauerkraut (fermented sauerkraut in a jar, never canned)
Coconut kefir (if you can find it)
Yogurt (plant-based, and avoid added sugars)

If you can't get what you need from your diet, are taking antibiotics, or need something more, do some research to find the right probiotics for you and your specific needs. A naturopath can also help you get you on the right path. Remember, the best time to take a probiotic is with the largest meal of the day.

BONE BROTH

If you want to do something really good for your health, it's time to listen up! Unless you've been sleeping under a rock, I'm sure you've heard about bone broth.

Bone broth is a broth made of bones that have been slow cooked for hours to get the gelatin and minerals out of the bone. You can make it at home or buy it from the store. Whichever you choose, make sure you start with grass-fed, pasture-raised beef bones if you're cooking beef bone broth, and free-range chicken if you're starting with chicken bones.

Bone broth is not the same thing as chicken, beef, or turkey broth. Look for the word "bone" in the title to make sure you're getting the right thing.

When those bones are cooked the right way, gelatin is released in addition to minerals such as vitamin K, calcium, phosphorus, and magnesium that are stored in bones. The gelatin is broken down into collagen, which is important for healthy teeth, thick hair, strong nails, supple skin, limber joints, and sealing gap junctions in the gut.

Here's more about this important material in your body.

COLLAGEN

Collagen, the most abundant protein in the body, is the glue that holds the body together. It provides structure, support, and strength to your skin, muscles, bones, and connective tissues. Collagen also plays a huge role in leaky gut healing and gut restoration.

Starting at age eighteen, collagen starts to decrease by about 1 percent every year. Of course, you don't see these changes right away, but eventually signs start to show. In addition, environmental factors such as smoking, stress, and diet increase collagen loss.

The result of plummeting collagen levels are aching joints, sagging skin, premature wrinkles, and decreased mobility.

It's difficult to get enough collagen from the modern diet. If you're not actively supplementing collagen, now is the time to start. That's why drinking bone broth and taking a collagen supplement are necessary. When purchasing collagen, I recommend getting a supplement with the five main types: types I, II, III, V, and X. In addition, for best results, make sure the collagen comes from sources that are naturally derived and uses grass-fed (when appropriate) and pasture-raised products.

Since vitamin C is needed for collagen synthesis, look for a collagen supplement that includes some vitamin C, or make sure you supplement vitamin C separately.

For best absorption, I recommend taking collagen in powdered form. Powdered supplements are better absorbed due to decreased particle size and can be easily added to drinks such as tea and smoothies, which makes taking them convenient.

Finally, be mindful of the expiration date on any collagen you purchase because nothing lasts forever.

DR. LISA'S NOTES

» Maintaining a healthy gut biome is an important aspect of immunity and overall health.
» Certain foods known as prebiotics feed good gut bacteria.
» Probiotics can be taken in the form of food or supplements to maintain a healthy gut.

WELLNESS PRESCRIPTION

» Pick two Be FINE probiotic foods to include as part of your meal plan this week.

NUTRIENTS

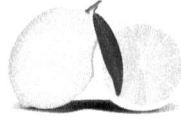

Chapter 19

MINERAL MASTERY

Micronutrient and nutrient deficiency are manifesting as disease, and you don't even know it.

It's time to talk about the "N" in the quest to be FINE. It's all about nutrients, and we're going to begin by exploring a few minerals that play a significant role in the quest for good health.

The body produces a select number of nutrients such as vitamins D, K, and certain B vitamins (thanks to gut microbes). Otherwise, vitamins and minerals cannot be synthesized in the body and need to be obtained from external sources. You owe it to yourself to maximize and optimize these nutrients safely.

There are two essential types of minerals: major minerals and trace minerals. The difference between them is that you need larger quantities of major minerals to keep your body functioning optimally. These minerals include calcium, chloride, potassium, sodium, sulfur, phosphorus, and magnesium. The body also needs trace minerals, but in smaller amounts. Some minerals in this group include chromium, selenium, copper, fluoride, iodine, molybdenum, manganese, and zinc.

It's important to know these minerals because a debilitating disease, a nagging condition, or a mystery illness could likely be the result of an underlying micronutrient or nutrient deficiency.

I'd love to tell you that to Be FINE you only have to load up on organic produce, eat pasture-raised/grass-fed protein, enjoy wild seafood, exercise, minimize inflammatory foods, wrap yourself in banana leaves, and say "cruciferous" three times, but it's slightly more involved than that. You can do all these things and still be sickly and micronutrient depleted.

In fact, dis/ease is often a result of nutrient and vitamin deficiencies. It doesn't matter if it is anemia, cancer, diabetes, hypothyroidism, or something else. If you can get to the bottom of what's causing the deficiency, you can often get to the bottom of what's ailing you.

Let's start by taking a closer look at daily recommended values (DRVs) of nutrients and supplements. A DRV is not the end-all-be-all, although people treat it as such. It is, however, a recommendation for the minimum daily amount of any vitamin or nutrient that the vast majority of healthy people should take based on gender and age.

The key words here are "recommended" and "minimum." The word *recommendation* tells you right away that these values are not individualized but rather a basic foundation.

Take me, for example. I had already freed myself from the likes of an impending autoimmune disease diagnosis, stopped eating foods my body found offensive, was maintaining a regular exercise regimen, and was eating nutrient-dense foods when I came face to face with my bathroom shower stall that tried to crack my head open in the wee hours of a cold Valentine's Day morning.

Soon after, I happened to be visiting my chiropractor and had my labs with me. It was only then that I came to the realization that my vitamin D levels were dangerously low. They were so low, in fact, that my chiropractor made a point to bring it to my attention. That alarm bell alerted me that since my vitamin D was out of sync, other vitamins, minerals, and nutrients could be in jeopardy as well. That idea led me farther down a rabbit hole of discovery, and as a curiosity-piqued student of life, I went happily down this tunnel.

You see, if your basement gets flooded, it's not enough for a water restoration company to just get rid of the water, check the sump pump, and repair the damage. What if the sump pump isn't the problem?

What if there are cracks in the foundation that led to the flooding? Or maybe you have a sump pump in your basement, but one sump pump is not enough or efficient enough to accommodate the water when it rains. Your foundation has to be repaired, or future floods will be likely and could be even more devastating. Those leaks may be slow at first, but eventually you'll see the paint on the walls start to swell. The carpet will start to get wet, and eventually you'll smell the stench of mold as it starts to grow.

You may not recognize that at first, but eventually the mold will make you sick.

Here's one of the common things I hear people say: "As I got older, my body started to change. I used to eat 'x' food all the time and never had a problem."

My response to these types of statements is always the same. Just because you don't *see* a problem doesn't mean you don't *have* a problem. In the human body, years of chronic stress, toxin exposure, and eating the wrong foods can lead to cracks in your foundation. It's like having an overworked sump pump. Eventually, leaks will occur and show up in places such as your skin, heart, gut, and joints. Toxic things will start to grow and make you sick.

Your foundation is important. And if you want to Be FINE, you have to go beneath the surface.

To go beneath the surface, you have to start with the gut.

IT STARTS IN THE GUT

As mentioned in Chapter 15, GMO foods, additives, artificial colors, toxins, pesticides, wheat, grain, allergenic foods, stress, and infections can all negatively affect the gut microbiome. That causes leaky gut and the malabsorption of nutrients. It's common to think that if you remove offending triggers and start eating right, then gap junctions will heal on their own. But it doesn't happen that way. A leaky gut doesn't naturally heal itself even with the avoidance or riddance of trigger foods and toxins. You have to do more.

Leaky gut syndrome has been linked with conditions and diseases such as food allergies and sensitivities, gut and bowel conditions (Crohn's, irritable bowel syndrome), psoriasis, arthritis, polycystic ovarian syndrome, and diabetes. In addition, holes in the gut can cause vitamin malabsorption and nutritional deficiencies.

To make things worse, foods such as wheat, grain, and legumes contain phytates. These molecules can bind to dietary minerals, including iron, manganese, and zinc, making those nutrients less absorbed by the body.

If you're already micronutrient depleted; if you're eating a heavy grain-filled diet; if you're feasting on conventional foods; or if you have gut disturbances, an autoimmune disorder, or a leaky gut, you can see why this would be a problem. (As you can see, when it comes to possible cracks in your wellness, the twin culprits of wheat and grain frequently pop up.)

While nuts contain phytates, they are great sources of nutrients such as magnesium, selenium, copper, vitamin E, fiber, and vitamin E.

So let's consider legumes for a moment. Legumes are a plant family that includes soybeans, beans, and peanuts.

Lectin is a plant protein found in legumes and has been said to bind to cell membranes, possibly causing inflammation in the small intestines. Lectins have been known to act as an *anti-nutrient*, preventing absorption of zinc, phosphorus, calcium, and iron.

Another important consideration is that lentils, which are a type of legume, have a high rate of cross contamination with crops such as wheat, barley, and rye.

Advocates of keeping legumes in the diet say, "Not so fast! If you cook the beans correctly, there won't be any problems."

Here's my take. The gut lining is only one cell layer thick and hence easily compromised. So it makes sense that up to 70 million people live with some type of gut disease. That number does not include gut intolerances or people who have yet to be diagnosed with a disease.

Also undisputable is that beans have been a staple part of the diet of many cultures for thousands of years and are highly nutritious. If you're currently healing or suffering from any gut intolerances, have micronutrient deficiencies, or are working on a gut-healing protocol, try removing legumes from your diet for ninety days, and see how you feel. That includes beans, peanuts, and coffee. These are all legumes!

If and when you're ready to reintroduce legumes such as lentils and legume-based pastas back into your lifestyle, make sure they are organic and free of major allergens such as gluten.

While the gut is one of the most regenerative organs in the body, the time it takes for your gut to heal will depend on your individual condition and any underlying conditions you may have. In addition, time is needed to bring down any inflammatory antibodies that may have developed.

During this time of gut healing, you should obviously still be focusing on Be FINE foods such as non-GMO organic produce, non-grain starches, wild fish, grass-fed meats, and pasture-raised chicken. You should be staying away from processed foods, dairy, and other triggers. Including gut-healing foods such as bone broth and homemade applesauce (with the skins) helps with restoration and healing. In addition, nutrients and supplements such as zinc, L-glutamine (an amino acid), eating probiotic-rich foods and adding a separate probiotic are very beneficial.

This is not deprivation. It's all about gathering information so you can learn more about your body and make informed decisions along the way.

VITAMINS, NUTRIENTS, AND MINERALS

Talking about nutrients is particularly important since many people are under the misguided assumption that they can get all the vitamins, minerals, and nutrients they need from food. Nothing could be farther from the truth.

Years ago, when I spotted a dime-sized bald spot in my hair, I thought I was getting all the nutrients I needed.

Due to modern farming practices and soil depletion, the fruits and vegetables of today are less nutritious than they were in the past. As a matter of fact, between 1950 and 1999, the USDA looked at the nutritional profiles of 43 fruits and vegetables, and what they found was quite surprising. There was a noticeable decline in minerals and vitamins, including calcium, iron, phosphorus, and vitamin B2 (riboflavin). In fact, studies have shown that over the last 100 years, the decrease in nutrients in our food is between 80 percent and 90 percent.

So what does this mean? Simply put, the spinach you bought from the grocery store (whether organic or not) is not as nutritious as the spinach your grandmother and your mother ate many years ago. You can load up on fresh, organic, non-GMO produce, get adequate exercise and sleep, and still walk around sickly and micronutrient depleted.

It happened to me, and it can happen to you.

Now let's take a moment and discuss some of the vitamins, nutrients, and minerals you need in order for your life to Be FINE. But before we move on, please remember that these nutrients are not a replacement for healthy eating and living a healthy lifestyle. They are an *enhancement* to it. Obviously, the nutrients I mention are not individualized, so you'll want to talk with appropriate wellness providers to see what you need.

If you have had bypass surgery, experience periods of high stress, have gastrointestinal disorder, are elderly, are raising kids, are reading this book, live on earth, or are breathing air, please note that micronutrient deficiencies are common and that simple multivitamin supplementation is not adequate to live healthfully well. To do that, you have to supplement, with food and likely through exogenous sources that are chemically extracted.

Supplementation can take place in different forms. Taking a pill is certainly one way, but you can't ignore that there is a bounty of foods that, when taken in the right quantities and preparations, can deliver clinical results.

Being the holistic food nerd that I am, later in the book you can expect to find a lot of food ideas on how you can get these nutrients.

Let's start by talking about a major mineral that 80 percent of Americans don't get enough of.

MAGNESIUM

Magnesium is one of those important minerals that just doesn't get the attention it deserves. Unfortunately, about 80 percent of people have low magnesium levels. It acts as a cofactor in more than 300 enzymatic reactions. They include blood pressure regulation, carbohydrate metabolism, energy production, heart regulation, stress, anxiety, and much more. A magnesium deficiency can also adversely affect other nutrients such as vitamin D and zinc.

Below are some symptoms of low levels of magnesium.

lightheadedness	shortness of breath	irregular heart rhythms (arrhythmias)
constipation	insomnia	fainting spells
migraines	seizures	tingling in the hands and feet
restless legs	muscle cramps	mood disorders and agitation

Think about it. How many people do you know who are affected by insomnia, migraines, or unmanaged stress?

Low levels of magnesium have specifically been linked to both stress and anxiety. It is one of the reasons that trips to the beach are so incredibly soothing. Magnesium, one of the minerals found in seawater, is both calming and relaxing. A pleasant visit to the beach goes beyond the fact that you are away from work and life stressors.

In the Caribbean, it's common practice for parents to take their kids to the beach, hoping they will be "knocked out" by the time they get in the car to ride back home.

The body also needs magnesium to regulate blood sugar. Low dietary magnesium is associated with insulin resistance and diabetes. In fact, magnesium supplementation is correlated with the prevention and management of diabetes and other cardiometabolic diseases.

But if you don't know what to look for, you won't know that hypomagnesemia (low magnesium) could be an issue. Unfortunately, magnesium levels are not typically accessed during routine annual doctors' visits. Even when they are, blood serum (extracellular) magnesium levels are often taken, which only represent 1 percent of magnesium levels. That is because 99 percent of the body's magnesium is intracellular and is found in bone, muscle, and soft tissue. Therefore, because it's so easy for low magnesium levels to slip quietly under the radar, serum magnesium levels are clinically less relevant when used as a tool to measure the body's magnesium levels. Severe hypomagnesemia can also cause hypocalcemia (low calcium) and hypokalemia (low potassium).

Could you be low in magnesium? Up to 80 percent of Americans are.

How Much Magnesium to Take

Supplementation is a very individual thing. So while I can't tell you how much magnesium you should take (if any), national guidelines vary for adults over age nineteen at 310 mg to 420 mg a day. Specifically, the recommendations are between 310 mg to 320 mg for women and 410 mg to 420 mg for men. Talk with a naturopath or functional medicine doctor to get more specific since those guidelines are not individualized, and in the case of magnesium, more is not necessarily better.

Magnesium Supplements

Should you choose to supplement, know that all magnesium is not created equal. The key is to pick wisely. Some options for supplementation are magnesium glycinate, malate, and citrate. Although magnesium citrate is easily absorbed by the body, it has a laxative effect.

Magnesium bicarbonate (not available as a ready-to-go product) can be easily made at home and tends to be more cost-effective than other types of magnesium available over the counter. Additionally, food or food-like sources of magnesium are better absorbed by the body. The recipe below for magnesium water is cost-effective and easy to make.

There are several recipes for magnesium water. Here's one that was shared by Dr. Williams Davis, author of *Undoctored*.

Recipe for Magnesium Water (Magnesium Bicarbonate)

Ingredients

2 liters unflavored seltzer water (seltzer water is just carbon dioxide and water; avoid tonic water or club soda)

3 tbsp unflavored regular Milk of Magnesia (MOM)

A large glass bottle (or several smaller glass bottles for storage)

Directions

Start with a 2 liter bottle of seltzer water. Remove 3 tablespoons, and discard.

Refrigerate the seltzer water for one hour.

Shake the MOM well.

Remove the cap from the seltzer water, and quickly add 3 tbsp (45 ml) of MOM (the less bubbles lost the better).

Shake well, and return to the fridge.

After 30 minutes, check again to make sure all the sediments are dissolved.

If the MOM you're using has 1,200 mg of magnesium hydroxide to start, each 1/2 cup (4 oz) serving yields 90 mg of magnesium. You can take up to 16 oz in two to four divided doses and get up to 360 mg of elemental magnesium per day.

Taking the magnesium this way yields less of a laxative effect and is easily absorbed, convenient, and easy to make.

Magnesium-Rich Foods

While supplementing magnesium is easy, I want to stress the importance of seeking out magnesium-rich foods and taking advantage of them as much as possible. Be FINE food sources of magnesium include almonds (opt for raw, not roasted or salted), pumpkin seeds, cooked Swiss chard, spinach, kelp, wheat grass, bananas, wild salmon, molasses, cucumbers, seaweed, raisins, and sprouted seeds. As a matter of fact, raw almonds have been my preferred snack food while writing this book. They keep me focused and writing.

The More You Know, the More You Glow!

Magnesium baths or soaks are a cost-effective way to get some of the magnesium you need. Since the skin is the largest organ of the body, magnesium bath soaks allow the magnesium to be absorbed. Soaking in a magnesium bath helps relax the body, soothe muscle aches, and prepare the body for a restful night's sleep.

Try This: A FINE Bedtime Bath Soak

Add 2 cups fragrance-free Epsom salt (magnesium sulfate) to running, warm bathwater, 3 drops of lavender essential oils, and 2 drops of ylang ylang essential oils. Soak in this fragrant magnesium bath for 20 minutes, and you won't have to worry about counting sheep.

If you don't have a tub, use one cup Epsom salt as a foot soak, or make a quick exfoliator you can use in the shower. To make the exfoliator, mix a couple tablespoons of Epsom salt with your favorite shower gel in a bowl or in your hands.

Magnesium is such an important nutrient. It's a shame that people don't know more about it. But now you do!

Whew! That section was jam-packed. You're more than welcome to stop and take a sip of coconut water here. It's full of electrolytes, including potassium, sodium, and—wait for it—magnesium.

CALCIUM

Like magnesium, calcium is one of the most important nutrients. Everyone needs it. But taking it is more than about building strong bones. Calcium facilitates the contraction of muscles, helps blood clotting, and keeps the heart, nerves, and muscles functioning optimally. Contrary to popular belief, when it comes to the best places to get calcium, you don't even have to wear a milk mustache to get it.

Be FINE sources of calcium include almonds, seeds (sunflower seeds and pumpkin seeds), and dark leafy greens such as kale, spinach, collard greens, and bok choy.

I'm not going to talk about calcium supplementation in depth since excess calcium can do more harm than good. If you want to address calcium levels, you have to be willing to learn about other nutrients since they affect calcium concentrations. For example, having too much calcium in the blood is antagonistic to magnesium absorption. Alternatively, having the right balance of magnesium inside the cell prevents calcium from causing possible damage. Therefore, the *ratio* of calcium to magnesium is more important than supplementing with calcium on its own.

In many cases, if you are taking a good multivitamin and getting adequate amounts of magnesium and vitamin D, you don't need a separate calcium supplement.

Dairy-Free (Be FINE Approved), Calcium-Rich Foods

Almonds
Broccoli rabe
Broccoli
Chia seeds
Dried figs
Fortified nut milk
Kale
Spinach
Sunflower seeds

The roles of calcium and magnesium are opposite in many ways. Look at the table below to get a better understanding of their roles in the body.

Role of Calcium vs. Magnesium

Role of Calcium	Role of Magnesium
Promotes blood clotting	Keeps blood flowing
Found mostly outside of cells	More intracellular (inside cells)
Excitability/contraction	Relaxation
Found in bones	Found primarily in bone and soft tissues

ZINC

Another mineral important for living a healthy and Be FINE life is zinc, which is utilized in more than 100 enzymatic reactions in the body. It's needed for immunity, maintaining gut health, healthy adrenal function, fertility, good thyroid function, wound healing, protein synthesis, collagen synthesis, healthy nails, thick hair, and more.

Zinc deficiency is also linked to gluten sensitivity.

Symptoms of zinc deficiency include leaky gut, impaired fertility, low immunity, slow wound healing, light sensitivity, memory loss, acne, hair loss, muscle atrophy (muscle loss), night blindness, and depression.

And those white spots you may have spotted on your nails have nothing to do with the number of boyfriends you have. Where does this folklore come from, anyway? White spots on the nails are yet another sign that you may have a zinc deficiency.

Since zinc is needed for protein synthesis, a deficiency can lead to balding, thinning of the hair, and brittle nails. Do you remember those tiny emerging bald spots that started to make their way in certain spots of my scalp?

Bingo!

Once you understand this, it makes sense why many alopecia patients have also been found to have zinc deficiency. So if you have been plagued by thin or balding hair, you want to make sure you're getting enough zinc.

Zinc should also be considered in the treatment of acne.

Storytime: For much of my teenage and early adult life, I was afflicted with terrible acne. One of the lowest points was when a dermatologist stuck a needle directly into my face in a weird attempt to get my face to "calm down." As many doctors as I saw and as many products that I tried, a nutritional deficiency was never mentioned during the doctors' visits or on any product labels.

Besides acne, other skin conditions such as dermatitis, rosacea, and eczema also benefit from adequate zinc levels. That can happen either naturally through food or with direct supplementation.

The use of birth control, eating a diet with little to no meat, using certain prescription medications, alcoholism, Crohn's disease, celiac disease, and anorexia are some of the risk factors for zinc deficiency.

Getting Enough Zinc

The current recommended dietary allowance of zinc is 11 mg for men and 8 mg for women. The fact that zinc is known as a trace element has nothing to do with its relative importance to wellness and well-being but everything to do with the small amounts needed to meet the recommended daily amount.

Remember, daily recommended values are not upper daily limits. Daily recommended values are also not the specific amount of any mineral or supplement needed to treat deficiencies, address acute concerns, treat infections, or optimize immune health. For example, the upper limit of zinc (amount you can likely take without encountering known harmful side effects) is 40 mg for both males and females.

Daily recommended values are a useful start. Work with a holistic clinician or functional medical doctor to find out what's best for you.

Seafood sources of zinc include oysters, crabs, and lobsters. Oysters lead the pack in terms of their zinc content with just three oysters providing more than 100 percent of the daily recommended value. But you don't need to eat raw oysters to get the zinc they provide. As a matter of fact, eating raw oysters can also expose you to bacteria, toxins, and heavy metals such as mercury and cadmium.

If you decide to get your zinc by eating shelled crustaceans such as crabs and lobsters, take note that I didn't say anything about having drawn butter, hush puppies, corn on the cob, and French fries on the side!

Grass-fed beef and lamb can also contribute to the overall levels of the zinc you need.

When it comes to plant sources, pumpkin seeds, hemp seeds, almonds, cashews, spinach, mushrooms, lentils, chickpeas, and cocoa powder are also good sources. Since our bodies do not store or synthesize zinc, it's important to get the correct amounts each and every day.

When it comes to anemia, most people just think about iron, but a zinc deficiency can also play a role in this condition that affects about two billion people globally. That's because a decrease or unavailability of trace elements, including zinc, can decrease iron absorption.

In addition to making sure you're getting the right amount of zinc, you should know that you get even more benefits from this nutrient when it's paired with a zinc ionophore (a complex that helps zinc ions get across fat soluble cell membranes). Zinc ionophores increase intracellular concentrations of zinc in the body.

One of the best-known zinc ionophores is quercetin. Capers are the best food source of quercetin. Other food sources of quercetin include raw banana peppers, dark grapes, elderberries, kale, onions, and apples. To get the benefits of quercetin in apples, you must eat the skin of the apples. This is yet another reason to shop and eat organic produce!

TWO NUTS A DAY KEEP THE DOCTOR AWAY

Apples are incredibly healthy. As mentioned above, they are packed with quercetin, have dietary fiber, and taste great. Apples also contain vitamin C, copper, and vitamin K.

When it comes to gut health, apples are packed with pectin, a carbohydrate found in high levels in apple skins. When apples are cooked with their skins, the pectin is more readily available. It forms a protective layer in the gut and acts as food for good bacteria.

Even with all this, you can get many more micronutrients from eating just two Brazil nuts a day.

Who knew?

Side by side, apples are less nutritionally equipped than Brazil nuts. These mega sources of nutrition are packed with micronutrients, including zinc, manganese, copper, vitamin E, vitamin B1, and selenium.

The daily recommended value of selenium is 55 mcg per day. Just two Brazil nuts provide a whopping 90 mcg of this important nutrient.

Don't go popping them like candy though. Due to the high selenium content, it's possible to get too much selenium and go into the toxic range. That's why it's important to not exceed three Brazil nuts per day and to snack and supplement appropriately.

The benefits of selenium are worth noting, and adequate levels are a vital part of the Be FINE plan. That includes prevention and improvements in cognitive decline, decreased incidences of cancer, reduction of oxidative stress, and hormone balance. The consumption of Brazil nuts has been related to an improvement in conditions such as dementia and Alzheimer's and when more focus and memory support are needed.

When it comes to hormone balance, the thyroid gland has the highest concentration of selenium than any other gland in the body. Not surprisingly, a very strong link has been shown between selenium deficiency and thyroid dysfunction. Hence, selenium supplementation through appropriate Brazil nut consumption is a potential option for people with decreased T3 thyroid levels.

If you've read this section and are wondering, "So, what's the bottom line? Should I stop eating apples?"

The answer is absolutely not!

Keep eating fresh, organic apples. They are delicious as well as nutritious. But make sure those apples come with one or two Brazil nuts on the side.

In the next chapter, I'll continue the discussion on minerals and also talk about a selection of vitamins you'll definitely want to make part of your wellness regimen.

DR. LISA'S NOTES

» Your body needs a combination of the right minerals and vitamins for optimal health.
» The lack of the right amount of nutrients in the right quantities is known as nutrient deficiency and is at the foundation of many diseases and conditions.
» Most people are not getting enough magnesium.
» Two Brazil nuts a day keeps the doctor away.

WELLNESS PRESCRIPTION

» Every day, eat one food that is rich in either magnesium, calcium, or zinc. Or eat foods that contain all three! (I won't mind.)

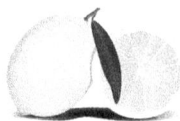

Chapter 20

VITAL VITAMINS

You have to be bold in order to shatter the chains of generational illness. Passivity is the deficiency.

VITAMIN C

Everyone knows about vitamin C, yet there's still much that is under-appreciated about this powerful vitamin. Getting adequate amounts of vitamin C goes beyond the avoidance of scurvy or amelioration of the common cold.

When it comes to nutrients, vitamin C is an important supplement you need to get enough of because the body does not make it on its own. To get what the body needs, you have to get it from food or supplemental sources.

But before you go stocking up on orange juice, you should know that food sources of vitamin C go beyond citrus fruits such as oranges, lemons, and limes. Cup by cup, there are other fruits and vegetables with even more vitamin C than oranges. Some of the highest and most accessible are kiwis, papayas, and bell peppers. If you live in Australia, you'll be delighted to know that the kakadu plum is the richest source of vitamin C in the world! The vitamin C content is 100 times more than oranges.

Other great sources of vitamin C–rich foods include mangoes, straw-berries, guavas, and black currants. For example, guava has four times more vitamin C than an orange, and a single serving of black currants contains a whopping 85 percent of the daily recommended value of vita-min C. Cruciferous vegetables such as Brussels sprouts and cauliflower are underappreciated sources of this powerful vitamin. And while one cup of cabbage only contains 30 mg of vitamin C, once it's fermented, traditional sauerkraut boasts an impressive 600 to 700 mg of vitamin C per cup! As a result, traditionally fermented sauerkraut is a probiotic superfood. Vitamin C is also found in foods such as broccoli and berries.

Speaking of berries, fruits such as buckthorn berry and amla are robust sources of vitamin C. Thankfully amla is a bit more accessible and affordable than the evasive kakadu plum. Frequently used in ayurvedic medicine, amla has been shown to reduce cholesterol and limit cancer cell growth. It also has powerful anti-inflammatory benefits.

As found in fruits like amla, vitamin C is also a powerful antioxidant that can provide immune support. In fact, high dose IV vitamin C has been used as a holistic adjunct to treat cancers and infectious diseases. Other benefits of the vitamin include increased mineral absorption, faster wound healing, and improved cardiovascular health. When it comes to bone and collagen health, vitamin C is essential, acting as a cofactor needed for collagen formation. And, while many think of calcium and vitamin D only when it comes to osteoporosis prevention, there is evi-dence that vitamin C supplementation also plays an important role in increasing bone density and reducing osteoporosis.

And since vitamin C is needed for collagen formation, its importance reverberates in keeping joints moving smoothly and minimizing the appearance of deep wrinkles. For skincare, not only is ingesting vitamin C important, but adding a vitamin C serum to your skincare regimen can help fight off free radicals to keep skin supple, reduce hyperpigmentation, curb acne, prevent sagging, and keep other skin ailments under control.

Like zinc, vitamin C plays a role in enhancing the absorption of iron. It does that by attaching to non-heme iron (iron that comes from plant sources) and making it more absorbable by the body. In fact, when eating non-heme iron sources such as spinach and kale, the addition of vita-min C–rich foods is known to enhance absorption. You can do that by squeezing some fresh lemon juice on a spinach salad, making a lemon vinaigrette, or enjoying a recipe like my sauteed kale with lemon.

When it comes to supplementing with vitamin C, many people fall short of what they need. Here's how to get the most from your vitamin C supplements.

Tips for Purchasing Vitamin C Supplements

The RDA of vitamin C (currently 90 mg for men and 75 mg for women) was determined by using the avoidance of scurvy as an endpoint. Scurvy is a disease caused by extreme vitamin C deficiency and characterized by bleeding gums, anemia, and weakness. It was often experienced by early nautical explorers who did not have access to fresh fruits and vegetables while on long journeys across the ocean. The solution was discovered in the eighteenth century by British naval surgeon James Lind who urged the Royal Navy to stock citrus fruits on board all its ships. British sailors soon earned the nickname Limeys among American sailors who didn't yet know about or believe in this effective treatment.

I don't know about you, but the mere avoidance of disease is not my idea of well-being. Vitamin C is necessary for things such as immunity, cardiovascular health, collagen production, wound healing, and minimizing free radical formation. Just reaching the RDA is barely scratching the surface in terms of optimal wellness. As a result, try to make sure you are getting at least 1,000 mg of vitamin C per day. That is still below the upper limit of 2,000 mg of vitamin C per day. If you are working with a holistic practitioner, experiencing active disease, or are on an immune-boosting protocol, it is likely that you will stretch those upper limits of vitamin C.

Ideally, optimum levels are achieved through food sources and whole food vitamin C supplements versus ascorbic acid. The ascorbic acid found in supplements is chemically synthesized and often derived from GMO corn, rice, and sugar. There is a growing body of evidence that shows that habitual use of ascorbic acid doesn't come without consequence. That includes but is not limited to lower exercise endurance and the depletion of copper. Copper is an important trace mineral needed for red cell formation, iron absorption, and bone and connective tissue building, as well as immune function and support.

When supplementing, your vitamin C supplement should also be gluten-free and dairy-free, and contain no monosodium glutamate (MSG) or soy. Ideally, whatever vitamin C supplement you choose will be free of added sugars as well.

VITAMIN D

Vitamin D is an essential fat-soluble nutrient that plays a pivotal role in keeping people healthy. It is synthesized by the body when bare skin is exposed to UVB (ultraviolet B) sunlight (cutaneous production), but can also be obtained through supplements or fortified food. Since humans can produce vitamin D, it is also considered a hormone. While there are thirteen essential vitamins the body needs, only vitamins D and K are capable of being produced endogenously (inside the body).

There are vitamin D receptors in almost every cell in the human body. That by itself should tell you something. Your body is intelligently and uniquely designed not only to produce vitamin D but to utilize it.

Although that is the case, it doesn't change the fact that about 80 percent of people are deficient in this crucial vitamin. Factors that affect vitamin D synthesis (production) include the following:

- Latitude (higher latitudes and greater distances from the equator result in decreased production)
- Altitude (solar UVB rays reach the earth more quickly at higher altitudes)
- Age (cutaneous vitamin D production decreases with advanced age)
- Air pollution (like ozone, reduces synthesis)
- Glass or plastic (UVB sunlight is greatly blocked by glass and plastic)
- Season (during the winter season in geographic areas above and below 33° latitude—far north and south of the equator—endogenous vitamin D production is greatly minimized)
- Sunscreen (use of sunscreen absorbs UVB rays, which is needed for cutaneous vitamin D production)
- Skin pigmentation (melanated skin has built-in natural sunscreen)

The role of vitamin D goes beyond increasing calcium absorption to keep bones and teeth strong. Vitamin D also plays an important role in maintaining immunity and muscle movement, decreasing inflammation, lowering mortality risk, decreasing disease, improving mood, decreasing depression, improving cognition, slowing premature hair graying, combating brittle hair, and helping you sleep at night.

If you think that's impressive, I've saved the best for last. Research has also shown that vitamin D improves cardiovascular risk, decreases incidences of both types 1 and 2 diabetes, increases immunity, diminishes the incidence of disease, and reduces cancer cell growth. You'll likely have to take more than the minimal intake of vitamin D to tap into those benefits.

An analysis using data from more than 100 countries showed a reverse relationship between UVB exposure and the occurrence of the following cancers:

Breast
Bladder
Endometrium
Esophagus
Kidneys
Lung
Ovaries
Pancreas
Rectum
Vulva

Basically, the more UVB sunlight people were exposed to, the less likely those cancers were to develop.

There was also a risk reduction correlated with sun exposure and Hodgkin's and non-Hodgkin's lymphoma. That is encouraging information since modern guidance is one-sided in its approach, often only sharing the possible negative ramifications of irresponsible sun exposure.

It turns out that vitamin D also plays a role in the development and occurrence of allergies, including food allergies, allergic rhinitis, asthma, and other allergic conditions.

Adequate serum vitamin D has also been shown to improve glucose metabolism. Inversely, low vitamin D concentrations are prevalent in those with type 1 and type 2 diabetes. Thus, there is significant benefit in maintaining adequate serum concentrations in people at risk and those with diabetes. In addition, having a serum vitamin D level greater than 40 ng/mL has been shown to decrease incidences of cancer by as much as 67 percent. Other diseases and conditions that benefit from adequate serum vitamin D are high blood pressure, heart disease, fibromyalgia, bone loss, and multiple sclerosis.

Signs of Vitamin D Deficiency

Signs of vitamin D deficiency vary but can include poor mood (depression), fatigue, weak immunity, bone pain, and frequent illness.

Thanks to great marketing, getting a milk mustache may be the first thing that comes to mind when you're thinking about how to get more vitamin D, but you can do so much better than that.

Hello Sunshine!

There is so much information surrounding sun safety and skin protection that many people have forgotten that sensible sun exposure is healthy and necessary for human health. Sensible sun exposure means safely exposing bare skin to the sunlight without burning the skin. You don't want to burn the skin since sunburns put you at increased risk of melanoma and non-melanoma skin cancer. After getting adequate sunshine (based on skin type), protect the skin from the sun using hats, light clothing, and appropriate sunscreen, if necessary.

Ancient civilizations respected the power of the sun. The sun's rays were used for everything from energy, warmth, and agriculture to scheduling the day's tasks. At one point, the focused energy of the sun was even used to cook.

Vitamin D is so important that our body synthesizes its own supply. Even so, most people don't get what they need to stay out of the deficiency zone. Individuals with brown and dark skin tones have more melanin in their skin and are particularly at risk.

Mindful exposure of bare skin to sunlight helps set the circadian rhythm, is disease-protective, and remains one of the best ways to get vitamin D. And it's free!

A Word about Vitamin D and UVB Radiation

Are supplements better than making your own vitamin D? The short answer is not necessarily. But supplements do have a place in your diet. That is especially true when it comes to climate, latitude, preexisting conditions, and age. Since vitamin D is a fat-soluble vitamin, one of the potential yet rare drawbacks of supplementation is toxicity from taking too much.

You can't make too much vitamin D from the sun because the body has a built-in checks-and-balances system and destroys excess vitamin D the body doesn't need.

Getting vitamin D from natural sunlight is as simple as it gets, but there are some guidelines to safely get sunlight for the purpose of vitamin D synthesis—the right way. And getting sunshine through your car window or the skylight in your bathroom will not cut it. That's because most plastic and glass windows block the majority of the kind of ultraviolet light that is needed to make vitamin D.

The sun produces three types of ultraviolet (UV) light: UVA (ultraviolet A), UVB (ultraviolet B), and UVC (ultraviolet C) rays. Only UVA and UVB light make it through the atmosphere to the ground, while UVC light is trapped in the ozone and never penetrates the atmosphere. Both UVA and UVB can cause burns, skin damage, and premature aging. The difference is that only exposure to UVB radiation can make vitamin D. To do that, you have to be exposed to sunlight at the right time of day.

The general amount of sun exposure needed for adequate production of vitamin D is between ten and thirty minutes on bare skin per day, without burning. Darker skin complexions need more.

The Fitzpatrick classification system, developed by Thomas Fitzpatrick, is a way to assess your complexion and ascertain the likelihood that you will burn with sun exposure.

Fitzpatrick Scale

Type I – Burns easily, does not tan

Type II – Tans slightly, burns easily

Type III – Tans well to light brown, can still burn

Type IV – Tans easily, slight risk of burning

Type V – Low risk of burning, tans easily

Type VI – Does not burn, tan is achieved quite easily

Time your sun exposure during peak sun, which is between 10:00 a.m. and 3:00 p.m. Solar noon, when the sun is the highest in the sky, correlates with the strength of UV radiation. Since UVB radiation is stronger during that time of day, it's the best time for vitamin D synthesis. Solar noon varies based on your location but also changes from day to day based on the earth's orbit around the sun and its tilted axis, which corresponds to the time of the year.

Depending on your skin tone and how easily your skin burns, adjust the time of sun exposure and the amount of unprotected time in the sun. Since your face is the most sensitive to sun exposure, opt to protect your face with a hat and sunglasses, leaving limbs and other parts bare until you have reached your individual exposure time, again without burning.

That is not the only way to get vitamin D, but it is certainly nature's preferred way. If you are highly intolerable to the sun's rays and want more sun, all hope is not lost. Here are a few things you can do to build up your sun tolerance.

How to Build Up Your Sun Tolerance

There are a few things that were a consistent part of my Caribbean upbringing and gave me an advantage when it came to improved sun tolerance. We're going to focus on the things you can change. Since none of us have a say on how much melanin our skin has, let's move on to the next item on the list.

Sun exposure. While most of us can't pack our things and move to a tropical climate, gradually increasing sun exposure will help build up your *solar callus*.

A solar callus is a gentle way to build sun tolerance through gradual and increasing sun exposure every day. Of course, you need to be mindful during this process and cognizant of burning, but it gets better and easier as you go. Consistent, sensible sun exposure increases skin thickness and sun tolerance, and decreases the chances of future burning.

The next thing you can do is supplement with cod liver oil. To my chagrin as a child, my mom routinely gave me cod liver oil. Adding cod liver oil to your regimen can help in a myriad of ways.

For starters, cod liver oil is jam-packed with natural omega-3 and vitamin A. It also has potent anti-inflammatory and anti-cancer benefits which improves sun sensitivity. Think of it as an internal sunscreen. Since this is a natural supplement, the benefit of improved sun sensitivity will come with consistent use.

In addition, cod liver oil contains some vitamin D that can count toward daily values. It also contains vitamin A and omega-3s, and both have potent anti-inflammatory and anti-cancer benefits. Cod liver oil is thus one of the most undervalued, natural, super-beneficial supplements you can add to your regimen.

Tips to Prevent Sunburns

While commercial sunscreens are one option, they're not the only way to protect yourself from burning. As a matter of fact, some chemicals in commercial sunscreens have been linked to cancer. It's incredulous to think that some sunscreens put people at risk of developing the very disease they're supposed to prevent.

To lessen this risk, use a website such as the Environmental Working Group (EWG), and source your sun protection responsibly.

Here are some other ways to reduce the risk of sunburn. Foods naturally high in polyphenols have been shown to improve the skin's resistance to sun damage. Polyphenols are phytonutrients found in foods with a plethora of health benefits.

Polyphenol-rich foods include the following:

- Red grapes (the polyphenols are in the skins)
- Tea
- Dark chocolate
- Black elderberry
- Rosemary
- Black olives
- Capers
- Thyme
- Blueberries

Other foods such as those rich in astaxanthin reduce UV skin damage. Astaxanthin is an antioxidant that comes from algae. Algae produce astaxanthin naturally to protect it from the sun. Humans get some of this sun protection factor with the ingestion of foods rich in astaxanthin.

Foods rich in astaxanthin include the following:

- Wild-caught salmon
- Krill
- Shrimp
- Trout
- Crayfish

Eating more of these polyphenol-rich foods along with wild seafood like those above will naturally increase your protection from the sun. For supplement support, make sure to get adequate vitamin D. Proper levels are needed for melanin synthesis. Adding a fish oil supplement with omega-3s will help to reduce inflammation and decrease the likelihood of burning while in the sun.

Here are some other things you can do for natural sun protection:

- Know your skin type. Use the Fitzpatrick scale for reference.
- Light-colored clothing can help protect your skin when you're outdoors for an extended period of time.
- A wide-brimmed hat is effective to protect the face and decrease the chances of premature wrinkles on its delicate skin.
- Eat more omega-3-rich foods.
- Time your sun exposure, and be mindful of peak sun exposure (usually between 10:00 a.m. and 2:00 p.m.) that is great for vitamin D synthesis but more likely to cause burns.
- Load up on antioxidant-rich foods.
- Consider adding wild-sourced cod liver oil as a supplement.

Food for Thought

When I was a kid growing up in the Caribbean, almost every day I spent hours in the hot tropical sun. I waited in the morning sun at the bus stop and walked the rolling hills after school in the bright afternoon sun. After I got home and did my homework, I met up with friends outside and talked and played for hours. I never got sunburns, but as I got older, I began to shun the sun when I learned of possible ramifications of unprotected, prolonged sun exposure.

The more I hid from the sun, the more my sun tolerance and natural solar callus *decreased*. As my accumulated natural protection dwindled, I increasingly relied on chemical sunscreens.

I'm not telling you to throw all caution to the wind and streak your neighbors in the mid-day sun. After all, there are other variables to consider, including skin type, prescription drug use, and skin sensitivity, all of which will affect your tolerance for the sun.

However, I will say that while there has been much attention paid to the potential harm of the sun, not enough attention has been put on the many important health benefits of mindful sun exposure. There are things that can be done to enjoy the sun safely.

Be FINE Food Sources of Vitamin D

- Cod liver oil
- Egg yolk
- Sardines

- Plant-fortified milks
- Wild salmon
- Mushrooms fortified with vitamin D such as morels and chanterelles

How Much Vitamin D to Take

Thanks to advances in nutrition labeling, it's easier to track just how much vitamin D is contained in packaged food and snack items. That was a move made by the U.S. Food & Drug Administration because Americans were consistently not getting enough.

By now, you must be wondering how much vitamin D or what type of vitamin D supplement to take. For optimal wellness, serum levels of this fat-soluble vitamin should be drawn at least twice a year—once in the winter and another in warm weather months if you live in a varied climate.

It's difficult to supplement adequately when you don't know where your serum levels are. When it comes to vitamin D supplementation, make sure you're getting vitamin D3 with K2. Vitamin D3 raises blood serum levels higher for longer, so it is preferred. Taking vitamin K2 along with vitamin D is important to make sure that calcium makes it to the bones and doesn't get deposited where it doesn't belong.

Non-supplement sources of vitamin K2 include organic grass-fed butter, grass-fed beef, and lamb.

While different entities may have differing opinions, one thing is for sure—anything less than 20 ng/mL of serum vitamin D is not good enough and puts you at risk for sickness and disease.

Ideally, levels should be between 40 ng/mL and 80 ng/mL. More recent studies point to optimal levels between 60 ng/mL and 80 ng/mL. Even those with just a small deficiency in vitamin D can experience depression. Levels above 40 ng/mL are associated with positive outcomes and lower risk for diseases such as type 2 diabetes.

When most people think about the benefits of supplementing with vitamin D, they think about things such as bone fractures and rickets. But high serum levels of the lipid solid vitamin have been beneficial in other conditions, including neurodegenerative diseases such as multiple sclerosis, neurological diseases such as Alzheimer's, gastrointestinal diseases, and much more. As a matter of fact, having a serum vitamin D level greater than 40 ng/mL has been shown to decrease cancer risk by more than 60 percent compared to levels of 20 ng/mL or lower. Breast cancer risk was lower in women with vitamin D serum levels greater than 60 ng/mL.

WEAK AGING

One of the biggest health risks in those ages sixty-five and older are unintentional falls. These falls are likely due to increased bone fragility and muscle loss that comes with age. Age-related muscle loss is known as sarcopenia. This disease occurs in 1 percent to 2 percent of all adults, beginning at around age thirty-five. Once you start losing muscle, take a fall, or get injured, it can be a slippery slope from there. It's hard to move around or exercise if you have been injured and are in pain. Added body weight with decreased mobility can lead to further wear and tear of joints and muscles. That can lead to increased incidence of disease.

I experienced an accelerated version of this type of muscle wasting firsthand. While pregnant and on hospital bed rest, in a matter of six weeks my muscles dwindled to the point that I could not even support my own body weight. I later fainted when my heart (also a muscle) could not accommodate the stress of walking a few feet from the hospital bed.

I admit to all this only to say that sarcopenia is no joke. This loss of muscle is a major reason for decreased independence in Western aging. The manual labor that used to be part of life well into the advanced years has been replaced by modern conveniences. You don't even need to get up to change the TV channel.

The good news is that sarcopenia can be minimized. One way is through appropriate resistance training and getting adequate vitamin D. Something called hydroxymethylbutyrate (HMB) also plays a role. I'll talk about HMB later, but first let's look at vitamin D.

Not only are increased serum concentrations of vitamin D associated with decreased muscle loss, but dynapenia (or loss of muscle strength) is correlated with low levels of vitamin D as well. The bottom line is to be mindful of your vitamin D levels if independence, vitality, and healthspan are important to you. You're reading this book, so I think I know the answer to that.

Of course, exercise and strength training are important factors too. Don't think you're going to just take vitamin D and start being a muscle master or maven!

Hydroxymethylbutyrate (HMB)

HMB is a metabolite of leucine, a branched chain amino acid and building block of protein. Since leucine is an essential amino acid, you can only get it from your diet or through supplementation.

Here's the wonderful part: Studies show that HMB supplementation not only increases fat loss but boosts muscle synthesis in both younger and older adults. Hence, adequate D3 levels, healthy protein intake, HMB supplementation, and resistance training may be the recipe for combating age-related muscle loss. Muscle tissue not only makes you stronger and fosters independence and confidence, but increased muscle mass can decrease the risk of type 2 diabetes, and muscle tissue actually burns more calories.

Now that's something to feel strong about!

The Domino Effect

Any Caribbean home has a pack of traditional dominoes in the house. And while slamming down domino cards in a game of dominos with my family was fun, as a kid I would much rather line up the dominoes in a long, curved-line design and then touch the first one and watch the swift fall of every domino in its path.

That's just how vitamins and nutrients are. They don't exist in a micro-cosm. That is especially true with vitamin D. When supplementing with higher doses of vitamin D, levels of magnesium, calcium, and K2 are also important and should be addressed. That's why eating a plethora of fruits and vegetables is so important. Any one fruit or vegetable contains other nutrients and vitamins that complement and balance the others.

VITAMIN B

Vitamin B confuses people because there are eight types. Most women are familiar with B9, known as folate (synthetically known as folic acid), due its significance in neural health during pregnancy.

Anyone concerned about hair and nail growth will be familiar with biotin (also known as B7). You'll see this vitamin in hair and nail growth vitamins.

Cobalamin (also known as B12) is important for cognition and nerve health. Since B12 is only naturally found in animal products, people who eat little to no meat, fish, eggs, or dairy are at risk for B12 deficiency. As a result, people in this group should supplement and eat foods fortified with vitamin B12.

Additionally, those who are pregnant or nursing, people with underlying medical conditions, and the elderly are at risk of being deficient. In healthy conditions, gut bacteria make select B vitamins in limited amounts.

MICRONUTRIENT TESTING

If you want to know where you stand when it comes to nutrients, micronutrient testing is a good idea. Partner with a naturopath or explore convenient third-party testing to know what nutrients you may need more of or are deficient in.

DR. LISA'S NOTES

» The body cannot make most essential vitamins, so they have to be taken through food and other exogenous sources.
» Vitamin C is a powerful yet underutilized antioxidant that comes from numerous sources.
» Sensible sunshine exposure remains one of the most efficient ways to "supplement" with vitamin D.

WELLNESS PRESCRIPTION

» Look at your latest lab values within the last year. What is your serum vitamin D level? Based on your most current value, work with a wellness practitioner to get your serum concentrations to at least 60 ng/mL within the next year.
» If you don't have your recent vitamin D levels, it's time to get them! You can get them through any reputable lab or healthcare provider. If your insurance won't cover the cost, that's a sign that they don't cover you. You can also get these levels by using at home lab test kits.

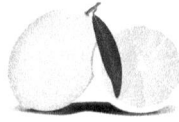

Chapter 21

INSIDE THE CARIBBEAN MARKET

If 74 percent of pharmaceuticals are derived from plants,
shouldn't we be teaching people about the plants that heal?

As a product of Caribbean ancestry, born and raised in the Caribbean, I'd be remiss if I didn't mention some of the nutritional gems hiding in your local Caribbean market. There are so many tropical fruits and vegetables that are jam-packed with vitamins. Here are a few of my favorites.

COCOA TEA

Do you remember that story I mentioned at the beginning of the book, about drinking cocoa tea as a child? Well, it turns out the cocoa tea made from natural cocoa is a nutritional powerhouse. That includes antioxidants and minerals such as vitamin C, vitamin E, and zinc.

TAMARIND

Have you ever heard of tamarind? You can't have a bite of this brown-shelled fruit without puckering up. It's like nature's Sour Patch candy except it's good for you. Just one cup of tamarind contains 92 mg of magnesium. But that's not all. In addition to all the other goodness, raw tamarind is also a good source of iron. Wrapped in a crunchy but inedible brown shell, tamarinds are packed with thiamine (B1) and magnesium.

CHRISTOPHENE

Next up on the list is christophene. Depending on where you are, some people also call this chou chou or chayote. This edible plant that belongs to the gourd family is packed with antioxidants such as quercetin and vitamin C. It has also been linked to improved heart health and reduced heart disease.

GUAVAS AND MANGOES

Other good sources of vitamin C are guavas and mangoes. For example, just three-fourths cup of mangoes contains 50 percent of the daily recommended value of vitamin C.

SOURSOP

Soursop has a green, prickly exterior but a sweet, white flesh. Soursops contain B vitamins, vitamin C, calcium, zinc, and more. It is one of my favorite fruits that grew in my yard when I was growing up. The problem was that the birds loved them even more! When it was time to pick the flavorful fruit, we often discovered they had already been devoured.

GUINEPS (KENIPS)

Believed to be native to the New World tropics, guinep is a fruit with several names: Spanish lime, quenepas, skinip, and mamoncillo. Besides potentially staining your favorite T-shirt, snacking on guineps will reward you with vitamin B and iron. If you've never tried guineps, they have the color of a lime on the outside with the texture of lychee fruit on the inside. They are quite remarkable.

GUAVAS AND BANANAS

When it comes to potassium, guavas and bananas are pretty hard to beat. Guavas contain 688 mg of potassium per cup, and bananas have 537 mg of potassium per cup.

SORREL

Growing up, I knew it was not officially the Christmas season until there was a pitcher of sorrel on the kitchen table. This drink, made from the red flowers of the hibiscus sabdariffa plant, is often confused with an edible green herb with an intense lemony tang, but these plants are totally different. Sorrel flowers have a blood-red color accompanied by a tart flavor similar to cranberries. Like the other items on this list, due to its affinity to warm and humid environments, sorrel is not exclusive to the Caribbean, but don't tell my family that. Some of the nutritional claims to fame are calcium, magnesium, potassium, and more.

The sugar in a traditional sorrel recipe is what you have to be mindful of. Monk fruit sweetener could be a worthy stand-in.

SEA MOSS

When I was a kid, sea moss was something I always heard locals talking about. So imagine my surprise when this ubiquitous species of seaweed, which grows abundantly in the turquoise waters of the Caribbean and along the rocky parts of the Atlantic Coast of Europe and North America, went mainstream, mentioned on every blog and health news outlet you could think of.

Why the booming interest? It turns out that sea moss, which varies in color from a greenish-yellow to red to dark purple or purplish-brown, contains 92 minerals of the 102 minerals the human body is made of. Some of these minerals are potassium, magnesium, manganese, chromium, copper, selenium, iodine, and many others you probably haven't heard of.

Speaking of iodine, there is considerable evidence that a deficiency in iodine is a modifiable risk linked to cancers of not just the thyroid but also the breast and stomach.

What's the point?

Eat your minerals!

The More You Know, the More You Glow!

Be FINE skin starts from the inside out. Make sure you're eating fresh fruits and vegetables that are high in vitamin C. Take a separate vitamin C supplement if your multivitamin doesn't have enough (most multis don't). By the way, vitamin C is such an important part of healthy skincare that you will find it as an ingredient in topical serums and lotions. Give your body what it needs to age healthfully well.

DR. LISA'S NOTES

» A plethora of vitamins and minerals can be obtained by eating a variety of produce—specifically, produce grown in warm tropical climates (such as the Caribbean), a gold mine for nutrients.

WELLNESS PRESCRIPTION

» Plan a visit to the produce section of your grocery store or (if you're feeling super adventurous) a Caribbean market, and try a fruit, vegetable, starch, or spice you've never tried before.
» For those already familiar with Caribbean produce, visit the ethnic aisle of your grocery store, a spice market, or an Asian or Indian grocer, and try a new spice or healthy food item you've been meaning to try or curious about. As with everything else, be mindful of ingredients, and make sure they are in alignment with the Be FINE lifestyle.

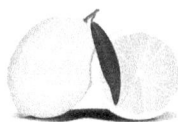

Chapter 22

INSIDE THE NATURAL
MEDICINE CABINET

Not all medicine is prescribed.

It's true—not all medicine comes from the pharmacy. If you're shutting your ears until you see it in an ad, until it's in a news segment, or until it's written on a prescription pad, your healing is no longer yours. You've outsourced it to a power outside of yourself that is more interested in profits than people.

You were made to heal from the inside out, not the outside in.

Do a little research, and you'll find that modern or conventional medicine became prevalent long after what we now call "alternative medicine." While modern medicine is about 200 years old, alternative medicine is 5,000 to 6,000 years old and was once considered common practice. So before we move on, let's first agree that we'll transition to using the terms "natural medicine" and "holistic medicine" whenever appropriate.

The pursuit of profits over people led to the standardization of medicine in the early 1900s, and things haven't been the same since. You see, nature can't be patented. Chemically developed entities can.

For example, while you can buy synthetically derived vitamin C as ascorbic acid, you can also easily walk into your kitchen and grab an orange to reap the benefits of natural vitamin C. So get ready! This "holistic pharmacist" has some things in her natural medicine cabinet that you'll want to add to yours.

BASIC SUPPLEMENTS LIST

There are some things you should always have on hand in your natural pharmacy just in case you need them.

After reading the chapter on nutrients, you may already know what to expect. If you're deficient in any of these nutrients, sickness and disease will knock at your door sooner than later. As a refresher, here are some of those vitamins and minerals, along with their preferred forms when indicated. We already discussed most of them in the nutrients chapter.

- Vitamin B complex
- Natural vitamin C
- Vitamin D3 plus K2 (softgels or liquid)
- Vitamin E (liquid or softgels)
- Fish oil (liquid or softgels – should come from wild-caught fish)
- Zinc

By no means is this an all-inclusive list.

In addition to a good multivitamin, the above list of vitamins and supplements will give you a running start on your Be FINE journey.

In addition to the minerals and vitamins listed in the Mineral Mastery and Vital Vitamins chapters, you can add other supplements to your Be FINE protocol as needed and appropriate. In many cases, you can look forward to lower incidences of cancer, a healthier heart, reduced inflammation, improved immunity, increased mobility, and firmer, more radiant skin. These supplements include but are not limited to the following:

- Collagen (types I, II, III, IV, and V)
- Resveratrol (found naturally in grapes and red wine) – anti-aging, antioxidant, and cardio-protective benefits
- Glutathione (known as the most powerful antioxidant) – made endogenously, but levels naturally decrease with age
- Black elderberry (provides immune support)

- L-glutamine (most abundant amino acid in the body) – levels can decrease with age. Supplementation can improve gut health, promote muscle growth, and help with leaky gut.)
- Curcumin (fermented or with black pepper for better absorption)
- Quercetin (reduces inflammation and risk of cancer)

TRIED AND TRUE HEALTH BOOSTERS

Apple Cider Vinegar

Apple cider vinegar is at the top of the list of tried and true health boosters because it's that important. It's produced by the fermentation of sugars from apples. The process creates acetic acid, which is full of anti-inflammatory benefits. Apple cider vinegar also contains important nutrients such as calcium, potassium, and magnesium. If the only time you think about vinegar is when you're cooking, you'd better think again.

I'm not talking about white vinegar. I'm not talking about those apple cider gummies with their blood-sugar-spiking ingredients of cane sugar and tapioca syrup. I'm talking about raw, organic, unfiltered apple cider vinegar—with the "mother."

The mother is the cloudy substance that settles at the bottom of the apple cider vinegar bottle due to fermentation. It's chock full of health enzymes. So be sure to shake the bottle before you enjoy it!

Apple cider vinegar is nothing new. It has been used for centuries—not just in cooking but as a natural medicine. Some of the documented benefits of taking apple cider vinegar include the following:

- Satiety or reduced hunger
- Blood sugar control
- Improved heart health
- Reduced belly fat
- Seasonal allergy relief
- Weight loss
- Lower blood sugar levels
- Improved digestion

To lean into these benefits, take 1 teaspoon to 2 tablespoons of apple cider vinegar in at least 8 ounces of water up to three times a day, ideally before meals. It's important that you take the apple cider vinegar diluted and not straight since it is highly acidic.

If you're just starting out, you can start at 1 teaspoon and work your way up. Take your first dose upon rising in the morning and then the remaining before meals for the rest of the day.

If you're fasting and using the fast friendly electrolyte recipe mentioned in Chapter 14, that would take the place of taking the apple cider vinegar in water as mentioned here. No need to use both.

EPSOM SALT

When I was a little girl growing up in the Caribbean, my mom was always ready to soak a body part in a bath of Epsom salt. I had my fair share of ankle sprains and twists while walking the hilly roadsides on my way home from school.

One of many naturally occurring mineral salts, Epsom salt is a compound of magnesium and sulfate found in rock-like formations. The name *Epsom salt* is a tribute to the town of Epsom near London, England, where the salt was supposedly discovered about 400 years ago.

Here's why Epsom salt is so beneficial: The magnesium in Epsom salt has been known to provide relief from everything from headaches, constipation, muscle pain, and body aches. Magnesium salts in Epsom salt are also beneficial in facilitating relaxation. So stock up. You'll want to have it in your home before you even need it.

HEALTHY NATURAL SALT

Long before people treated salt like it was kryptonite, salt was greatly revered. Salt and its uses date back to ancient civilizations. Used in everything from currency to religious ceremonies, there's a reason that Jesus's followers were referred to as "the salt of the earth" in the Bible.

When I discuss salt, I'm not talking about commercial table salt. That stuff is highly processed, has been stripped of healthy minerals, and is often bleached before being packaged for consumers. These salts are heavily added to processed foods and can wreak havoc on your health.

Ancient salts such as Himalayan salt, Maldon salt, and Celtic salt are minimally processed compared to table salt. These salts contain higher amounts of minerals such as potassium, calcium, and magnesium.

From a well-being perspective, salt is necessary for cellular function, adequate hydration, and proper electrolyte balance. As a matter of fact, when it comes to essential components of bodily function, salt is right up there with oxygen, water, and potassium.

Salt also has bactericidal properties that can be quite beneficial in keeping bad bacteria at bay. What's the point? The human body needs salt to survive.

"But isn't salt bad for you?" ask some people.

Here we go.

Similar to the fat-free fallacy, the vilifying of salt is yet another area of wellness that is misrepresented and misunderstood. Maybe I should call this the "salt-free fallacy."

The "salt causes hypertension idea" or "guilty by association theory" (as I like to call it) started almost fifty years ago. Current analysis questions this position and shows that people with low salt intake are actually at a *higher* risk of cardiovascular events due to increased cholesterol and insulin resistance.

I can hear you now: "So why is it that when I lower my salt intake, my blood pressure goes down?"

First, if you're only reducing salt and continuing to eat the SAD (standard American diet), these results will not be long-lasting. It's not like you're sitting down to eat bowls full of salt by itself. The salt was nestled in refined carbs, excess sugars, and processed foods.

When you limit these added salts, you also lower the amount of processed foods you're consuming. Lower carbohydrate intake means lower insulin levels since the body needs to produce less of it to keep blood sugar balanced.

Less insulin means the body flushes out extra water and sodium, which decreases blood pressure.

So here's the bottom line about salt and hypertension.

Highly processed foods are not just high in sodium but are also loaded with refined carbs, which indirectly elevates blood pressure.

Highly processed foods are low in potassium, which is not desirable because potassium helps reduce blood pressure.

Lowering refined sugars, getting adequate potassium, and keeping carbohydrates in balance are key determinants in lowering high blood pressure.

Focus on eliminating refined carbohydrates, packaged foods, and processed sugars. Foods that come from a plant or tree or from the farm contain very little sodium. You should be eating natural, salt-free foods to which you add your own healthy salt.

Now that we've gotten that part out of the way, once you've removed the processed foods, refined carbohydrates, and sugary foods, here are some ways to use unrefined salt.

Be FINE with Salt

Mouth rinse: Add ½ tsp unrefined salt to warm water, and swish in your mouth. Do not drink it. Spit it out after swishing. This is a cost-effective way to reduce bad bacteria, fight bad breath, and limit cavities.

A similar rinse can be made and used for gargling for sore throat relief. Again, do not swallow it. Be sure to spit out all the water after gargling.

Hydration: Dehydration is a culprit in many conditions, from headaches to seasonal allergies and other types of ailments. Salt helps water move into cells for adequate hydration.

Individuals with heart or kidney failure should consult with their primary doctor or wellness team before adjusting salt intake.

When I was a practicing pharmacist, I took an oath to give the right drug to the right patient at the right dose at the right time. I think of food and all-natural medicine in the same way. Using the right foods in the right dose at the right time along with ingesting the right foods is an integral part of your holistic wellness journey.

It's not about vilifying salt. It's about using the right salts in the right way while keeping other minerals in harmony.

Salt smartly.

MANUKA HONEY

Ohh . . . honey! I have something really sweet to tell you.

If you have a cough or itchy throat, Manuka honey is great at coating the throat, and it's full of inflammation-reducing agents that will get you back up to speed. Manuka honey is expensive compared to local or processed honey because it is produced by bees native to New Zealand.

These bees pollinate a specific flowering tree that blooms only two to six weeks of the year. Manuka honey is considered medicinal due to its antibacterial, antiviral, and anti-inflammatory properties.

In addition, the valuable sweet sap is useful for gut health and wound healing.

How to Buy Manuka Honey

Make sure the Manuka honey you're buying is from New Zealand. The label should also carry the Unique Manuka Factor (UMF) label and trademark. The UMF number should be between 10+ and 25+. The higher the number, the more nutritionally sound and expensive the Manuka honey will be.

UNSULPHURED BLACKSTRAP MOLASSES

It turns out that sugar is not all bad. As a woman of Caribbean descent, I take particular interest in this next item since sugar plantations were historically and economically important on the islands. There are different types of molasses. Blackstrap molasses is the darkest, thickest, and most nutrient-dense.

Considered a waste product of sugarcane processing, blackstrap molasses contains the least amount of sugar of the different types of molasses. Vitamins, antioxidants, and minerals such as vitamin B, zinc, potassium, manganese, selenium, phosphorus, calcium, and copper are packed in every spoonful. Blackstrap molasses is also an excellent source of non-heme iron.

In case you're wondering, that makes blackstrap molasses far more nutritious than refined sugar.

While consuming molasses in large quantities is not recommended due to the glycemic index, taking one tablespoon of molasses diluted in milk, water, or tea can act as a nutritional boost and may be beneficial in conditions such as iron deficiency anemia, fibroids, and heavy menstrual bleeding. Just one tablespoon of blackstrap molasses contributes 20 percent of the daily recommended value of iron. Blackstrap molasses can also act as a natural stool softener.

Use blackstrap molasses between meals. I don't recommend taking it straight up. It may not be for you if you have blood sugar issues or are trying to lose weight.

Storytime

For two years on and off, I had annoying foot pain that would not go away. I hadn't injured myself and could not determine the source of the pain. After seeing a chiropractor for more than a year to rule out alignment issues and getting no results, I decided to see a podiatrist. The podiatrist offered to fit me for special support shoes. While I knew that the shoes would likely help me feel better, this was not the source of the problem, so I declined.

Let me make this clear. I have nothing against orthopedic or support shoes. I just have an issue with orthopedic shoes *on my feet*.

On a whim, I started to supplement with blackstrap molasses. Within two days, the pain I had for two years disappeared.

Did you read that? The symptoms that I had for two years disappeared in two days.

Is this story cleverly inserted to convince you to take blackstrap molasses?

Maybe but, not necessarily.

I don't know your situation or your medical history.

Yet still, you have to admit that it was a pretty powerful story.

(Don't ever miss an opportunity to tell a powerful story.)

Diseases and ailments are often the symptoms of unknown nutritional deficiencies.

HYDROGEN PEROXIDE

There is no reason why you shouldn't have several bottles of hydrogen peroxide in your house at any given time. It's good for everything from cleaning small scrapes, mouth cleansing, and ear wax removal, and can be used as an antiseptic. The best part is, after all these years, generic hydrogen peroxide is still quite affordable.

CHARCOAL TABLETS

My first introduction to activated charcoal came decades ago when I worked as a pharmacy technician. Growing up on an island, fish, of course, was a staple part of the diet. But no matter how careful people were, it was inevitable that sometimes there would be a case of "fish poisoning."

That's when people came to the pharmacy and asked for activated charcoal. Activated charcoal works by binding toxins and chemicals in the body, preventing the body from further absorbing them.

When is the next time you'll encounter a toxin? That's the thing—you never know. No one plans for these things.

ESSENTIAL OILS

If you haven't tried essential oils yet, now is a good time to get on board. Essential oils have been around a long time.

Just how long?

Essential oils have been part of natural healing since biblical times. As a matter of fact, the three wise men journeyed to the manger with essential oils, including myrrh and frankincense, to greet the newborn baby Jesus. Queen Cleopatra used essential oils as part of her beauty regimen.

The point is that essential oils are not new to natural medicine, but it's okay if they're new to you. From using them as insect repellents or even as a tool to boost immunity, there is so much to learn and love.

I admit that it can be a lot. Your best bet (if you're just starting out with essential oils) is to buy a kit with just a few oils. You can also steal this list of favorites for wellness and immunity and make them your own.

Lemon Oil

Lemon essential oil is a natural antibacterial, anti-inflammatory, and detoxifier. By fighting bacteria, reducing inflammation, and detoxing the body, lemon essential oil also boosts the immune system. In addition, lemon is a natural disinfectant and can be used as a cleaning product. While this last feature doesn't bolster the immune system, it does help you reduce bacteria in the home and make it smell good.

Cinnamon Oil

Cinnamon oil is both an antibacterial and an antioxidant that helps boost the body's natural defenses against germs and bacteria. While cinnamon is known for its heart protective and insulin sensitizing effects, cinnamon oil is touted for its analgesic, antiseptic, antibacterial, anti-inflammatory, antifungal, and circulatory benefits.

Tea Tree Oil

Tea tree oil is one of the most versatile essential oils for the immune system. This oil has antimicrobial, antibacterial, and antibacterial properties. It's also an effective decongestant and expectorant, helping keep sinuses and airways free of gunk. In addition, used topically, tea tree oil can treat coughs, chest congestion, acne, and even cold sores.

Eucalyptus Oil

Like tea tree oil, eucalyptus supports respiratory tract health and is a natural decongestant and expectorant. There are more than 500 types of eucalyptus trees, but only three varieties are used to create eucalyptus oil.

Peppermint Oil

Peppermint is one of the most used essential oils. It relieves headaches, detoxifies, and is soothing to the respiratory system. In addition, this essential oil has antibacterial, antiviral, and anti-inflammatory properties. All this combines to make it a powerhouse among essential oils that also boost immunity.

Oregano Oil

Oregano is as good for your body as it is for your taste buds. While most people think of oregano as an ingredient in spaghetti or pizza sauce, the essential oil made from this herb is incredibly powerful. Oregano oil fights bacteria, viruses, and other microorganisms, making it an excellent oil for keeping your body healthy. Oregano oil has shown activity against small intestinal bacterial overgrowth (SIBO), reduced antibacterial resistance, and more.

The oil is also very concentrated, so be sure to use it sparingly.

Lavender Oil

Lavender is commonly used to help relieve stress and promote relaxation. Lavender oil is also rich in antioxidants and has antiviral, antimicrobial, antiseptic, and antibacterial properties. All these characteristics help boost immunity.

Rosemary Oil

Rosemary is a natural decongestant and expectorant, and helps your body expel any gunk that has built up in the airways. Rosemary oil has antibacterial, anti-infection, antifungal, and analgesic properties that help promote a stronger immune system. Regular inhalation has been shown to reduce stress and boost immunity. Rosemary oil is a great addition to do-it-yourself hair conditioning and helps invigorate the scalp for healthy hair growth.

Ylang Ylang

Ylang ylang will quickly become one of your favorite essential oils. First, the scent is amazing. Second, just a few drops do the body good. Whether you mix it with your favorite carrier oil and apply it topically or put it in a diffuser, the benefits can't be ignored.

Ylang ylang promotes relaxation, reduces anxiousness and nervousness, lowers blood pressure, and is an aphrodisiac.

Don't forget—the best medicine cabinets are well-stocked before they're needed.

By the way, if you're wondering how to pronounce it, it's "ee-lahng ee-lahng," but many Americans just say "lang-lang."

DR. LISA'S NOTES

» What's called "alternative medicine" is not actually alternative at all. The mischaracterization is a conscious effort to discredit natural medicine that has been around since the beginning of time.
» Everyone needs a well-stocked natural medicine cabinet. Stock it before you need it!

WELLNESS PRESCRIPTION

» Go to the list of items under "Tried and True Health Boosters" in this chapter. Use it as a baseline to begin stocking your natural medicine cabinet.

ELIMINATION, EXERCISE, AND ENERGY

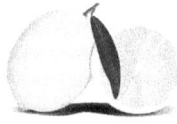

Chapter 23

ELIMINATION

You may think you're smart, but your body is smarter.

Do you remember that mindset shift I told you would be necessary to push through the hard stuff and make the changes you need to Be FINE? You're almost there. But to get to your reward at the end of this journey, first you have to learn how to eliminate.

Eliminate all you thought you knew about staying healthy.

Eliminate the idea that your doctor knows it all.

Eliminate the notion that if something "runs" in your family, you can't run past it.

Eliminate the idea that prescription medication is always better than natural medicine.

What deep-rooted thoughts or ideas do you need to eliminate when it comes to your health? Pause and write them below.

_____
_____
_____
_____

THAT'S SUCH A WASTE

Do you ever pause and marvel at how uniquely equipped your body is? It's actually pretty fascinating. Every intricate detail has been mapped out and considered ahead of time. One of those details is waste management.

Fortunately, you don't ever have to bundle anything up or take it out on trash day. Your only responsibility is to move more than you sit, eat right, get proper nutrition, and drink water.

DON'T WATER THIS DOWN

Drinking water is an important and often neglected part of wellness. I'm not talking about drinking coffee, tea, sodas, smoothies, or some fancy electrolyte drink. Good clean "sky juice" (as I like to call it) is what you should drink. Drinking adequate water is not just important in the summer but all year long.

Here are some things you should know about sky juice before your next water break.

- Decreases histamine levels (of great importance especially during allergy season)
- Regulates body temperature
- Fights fatigue
- Aids in the absorption of nutrients
- Helps fight illness
- Increases pain threshold
- Flushes bodily waste

How Much Water to Drink

We've all heard that you should drink eight cups of water a day. While that number is a good place to start, it doesn't take into account specific lifestyle variables such as weight and activity level. A more specific water goal is to drink two-thirds of your weight in water daily, on a scale of pounds (body weight) to ounces (water).

For example, if you weigh 150 pounds, you should drink approximately 100 ounces (or 12 to 13 cups). As a reference, one gallon is 128 ounces (16 cups) of water.

You may also need to drink more water based on your activity level.

When the body is adequately hydrated, it can eliminate waste more efficiently. This elimination happens through organs such as the kidneys, colon, lungs, and skin.

Urine (Kidneys)

One of the ways waste removal happens is through the kidneys by way of urination. Urine should be pale yellow, almost colorless. At no point should your urine be the color of Tang (that commercial breakfast drink) or school bus yellow.

The shade of urine is not only an indication of how concentrated it is but how hydrated you are. It tells you if you've been doing a good job of drinking water. Remember, the general guideline is that you should be drinking about two-thirds of your body weight in water each day on a scale of pounds (body weight) to ounces (water).

In addition, be sure to divide your daily water intake into several servings throughout the day. There's no "one and done" when it comes to drinking water.

Some Things That Affect Urine Color

While pale to amber urine is the gold standard, there are other factors you should be aware of that can affect urine color.

Diet

Foods such as beets, berries, carrots, rhubarb, and fava beans can affect the color of urine.

Medication

Both prescription and nonprescription medication can affect urine color. So be mindful, and always look in the toilet after you go.

Menstruation

If you are menstruating, that can affect the color of your urine.

If your urine has changed in color for unknown reasons and doesn't appear normal in color, be sure to consult a trusted member of your wellness team.

OH CRAP! (YOUR COLON)

It's a dirty job, but we all have to do it. And since my desire for you is to live a more healthy and vibrant life, this aspect is no different. When you gotta go, you gotta go. And by all means, I hope you're going.

At this point of the book, I'm assuming that you're eating lots of organic fruits and vegetables, getting adequate fiber, and drinking lots of water (two-thirds of your body weight in ounces) throughout the day.

These factors set the foundation for healthy bowel movements. Once you're there, here are four things to consider: shade, shape, smell, and schedule.

Shade

When I say shade, I mean color. The only way to know the color of your poop is to look in the toilet after you poop.

Seriously.

It's your responsibility.

Poop should be brown on most occasions. But other colors can make their way into the toilet bowl as well. If you see other colors, it's important to know what they could mean.

Green Stool

Green stool could mean diarrhea. Seeing green in your poop could also be a result of something you ate. For example, artificial dyes and lots of leafy greens could cause you to see green in the toilet.

Gray or Clay-Colored Stool

Yep. That's not a typo. Poop can be gray or clay-colored. If you see this color after going number two, it could be that there is a lack of bile in your poop. That could also happen if you're taking certain medications or if you have liver disease or another serious condition.

Red or Reddish Stool

As you can imagine, seeing bright red poop can be quite alarming. Foods such as beets or those that contain red dye could be a trigger. If you have eliminated your diet as a source of red poop, here is something else to consider. Consistent red or reddish poop could mean there is bleeding in the lower gastrointestinal tract. Don't wait—see a trusted health professional.

Yellow Stool

Yellow poop could mean there is fat in your stool. Fat in your poop is a sign of malabsorption and is a possible sign of a disorder. Yellow stool could also be a sign of a high-fat diet or the ingestion of food dyes. If your poop floats, that's another sign of high fat content.

Black or Tarry Stools

Black or tarry stools could be the result of bleeding in the upper gastro-intestinal tract and is a serious consideration. Other possible causes are the use of anti-diarrheal medications containing bismuth subsalicylate, iron supplements, and charcoal tablets.

Shape

Yes, stool should have a shape. And when it comes to what's dropping in the toilet, the Bristol stool chart says a snake-like or sausage poop is what you're looking for. Round pellets mean you're constipated. Blobs of stool that have no shape mean diarrhea. What you're looking for is poop that takes a nice Olympic dive versus several tiny splashes.

Smell

Unless we're talking about the poop from an exclusively breastfed baby, let's face it, the poop from other humans stinks. I mean poop is waste, bacteria, and things your body wants to get rid of. Essentially, the smell is one of the reasons we call it "taking a dump." Sitting on that toilet means you're taking out the trash.

As far as I know, trash doesn't smell like fragrant mangos at the peak of ripeness. It smells pretty unpleasant. The important thing to note is what smells are normal for you and if those smells change based on what you eat.

For example, foods such as peppers, garlic, and beans are notorious smell-shifters and may change the way your poop smells. Bacterial infection and diarrhea can do it too. The bottom line: pay attention to how your poop smells.

Schedule

Now that you have an idea of what your poop should look and smell like, it's time to talk about how often you should go. Most sources will tell you that pooping is a very individual thing and that no two bodies poop alike.

While that is true, there are some guiding principles. Ideally, you should have two to three good bowel movements per day with normal shade, shape, and smell. Minimally, you should be pooping at least once a day—none of that once-a-week nonsense.

Having a good poop schedule allows you to clear the colon, expel waste, and minimize toxicity that can otherwise manifest in illness.

If you're challenged with producing two to three good bowel movements per day, here are some things that can help you get there.

Gastrocolic Reflex

Gastrocolic reflex is a physiological response that causes increased gastric motility immediately after a meal. Basically, after you eat, the colon increases its movement as a response to food entering the stomach. That reflex is also very active in the mornings, typically within 30 minutes of awakening.

So if you can work with your body in the morning or after meals when it naturally wants to get the poop moving, that's a great time to go! If you tend to have busy mornings, wake up 15 minutes earlier, and allow yourself some time to go.

After meals, the gastrocolic reflex is responsible for increasing the food capacity of the stomach by pushing previously ingested food toward the rectum for expulsion. This not only allows room for food but is an opportune time to prioritize using the bathroom.

Poop Environment

If you're having a hard time pooping, it could be due to your poop environment. Music, a noisy environment, or tinkering on your phone during potty time (hello, I see you) are not giving your body the devoted time it needs to relax and get the poop out. If you work outside the home during the day, you can probably try pooping before work in the morning and after dinner when you get home where the environment is more familiar. If you decide to have bean burritos with your coworkers for lunch, I can't help you there.

Remember, your poop environment is only one aspect of good poop and gut health.

PROBIOTICS

As extensively covered in the gut check chapter, probiotics are a beneficial addition to any wellness regimen. Living bacteria and yeast can be taken in the form of food or supplements for the purpose of attaining better gut and overall well-being. Besides improving your health, probiotics can help bowel regularity, reduce diarrhea, and minimize intolerances to foods such as legumes and cruciferous vegetables. Probiotics are also beneficial in the metabolism of carbohydrates, protein, and fats.

BREATH (LUNGS)

The act of breathing is yet another way to detoxify. Since you've been breathing all your life, that may seem rather simple. The truth is, however, that most people don't breathe correctly. Breaths should be long and deep versus shallow and quick. Pranayama, which is a major component of yoga, can help improve your breathing.

The reason proper breathing is important is because the body expels waste through the lungs in the form of carbon dioxide. That happens through the mouth and nose during respiration. For that reason, whenever both your mouth and nose are covered, you compromise detoxification and healing.

Let me say it again for the people in the back. Whenever both your mouth and nose are covered, you compromise detoxification and healing.

SWEAT (SKIN)

Another way the body detoxifies is by excretion through the skin in the form of sweat. That can happen through exercise or other forms of exertion. Exercise or movement is a necessary part of the Be FINE lifestyle. It doesn't matter if that exercise happens in a gym, outside at a park, or inside your home. The important part is that you get moving and increase your heart rate. Don't forget to add weight resistance to your routine.

Treadmills are convenient but not a necessity. A bike ride with your kids, a riveting dance with friends, roller skating, or a walk around the neighborhood can all count toward getting your heart rate up and letting the sweat flow.

A study has also shown that just 25 minutes in a sauna has benefits that are similar to a moderate exercise session. Now that's something to get "excercited" about.

DR. LISA'S NOTES

» The body eliminates waste mainly through urine, feces, breath, and sweat.
» There was a lot of crap discussed in this chapter. I hope you were offended. I'm not going to make things weird, but the next time you sit on the toilet, don't forget the four S's: shade, shape, smell, and schedule.

WELLNESS PRESCRIPTION

» Set aside enough time to poop every day. Come on, you have to take the trash out. Once you go, look in the toilet. A healthy body produces healthy poop.

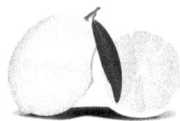

Chapter 24

EXERCISE (MINDFUL MOVEMENT)

Wellness visits don't happen once a year; they happen every day.

Getting into the habit of exercising is not always easy. That is especially true if you weren't a child athlete or didn't establish a habit of exercise in your younger years. You may feel like you don't have time or just don't like movement. If none of that applies to you, that's awesome! For everyone else, keep reading.

Not only is it important to find something you enjoy doing, but being mindful about how you can keep motivated will serve you well.

Here are some mindful movement motivators to get you inspired.

MINDFUL MOVEMENT MOTIVATORS

Exercise + Music

No matter what type of exercise you choose to do, you can pair it with music. It doesn't matter what type of music you like. Just put the music on, and get moving. Setting up an exercise playlist is also quite efficient.

Exercise + Play

If you're having a hard time getting or staying motivated to exercise, especially when it comes to cardio, try making it more playful and fun. Here are some exercise ideas that can also count as play.

- Skating
- Bike riding
- Tennis
- Jumping rope
- Swimming
- Trapeze class
- Pole dancing

Exercise + Nature

Exercise plus nature goes double duty because not only will your body get the benefits of exercise, but the benefits of being out in nature can't be beat. As a matter of fact, just a twenty-minute nature walk has been shown to reduce cortisol (stress hormone) levels. In addition, improvements in mood, mental well-being, and cognition have been connected to spending time outdoors. Spending two hours outdoors or in green spaces each week is associated with increased health and well-being.

Below are some other benefits of spending time in nature.

- Increased creativity
- Enlivened senses
- Change of scenery
- Boosted immunity
- Reduced blood pressure
- Plus . . . it feels good!

If you want to find more ways to incorporate nature into your exercise routine, here are some ideas to get started.

- Nature walks
- Surfing
- Swimming
- Hiking
- Skiing
- Gardening

- Taking outside whatever exercise you already do inside

Exercise + Competition

Not everyone is competitive. But if you are, you might as well use it to your advantage. Some things you can do include setting up a low-key, friendly contest with like-minded friends or colleagues for things such as body fat loss, number of days at the gym, or pounds lost. That may serve as the initial jump-start you need to keep consistent during your exercise regimen.

Here are some other ideas for pairing competition with exercise.

- Marathons
- Iron man/woman competitions
- Competitive swimming
- Contact sports (basketball, tennis, volleyball, etc.)
- Roller derby team

Exercise + Companionship

Not everyone likes being around or talking to other humans. But for those who do, these ideas for mindful movement may work for you. By the way, we all have our people. Even if you're not generally a people person, there's probably one person you like spending time with. See if this can work to your advantage and get you moving.

Below are some ideas for pairing companionship with exercise.

- Group exercise classes
- Pairing a phone call with a walk
- Exercise date: meet up with a person or people you like for the purpose of spending time together while you exercise.

Exercise + Community

Do you like being part of communities? I don't mean hanging out with people you already know and love. I mean being associated with or hanging out with people based on a common interest, whether in person or online. It could be based on religious affiliation, a hobby, where you work, a group of parents from your kids' school, or simply because you all want to lose weight.

Community is a powerful tool that can be leveraged for better health and well-being. If you thrive on a strong sense of community, you should seek out in exercise groups that are not only about the exercise routine but the built-in community you get with it.

If community is an important value to you, look for ways to integrate community in your fitness regimen. It will be an integral part of your success.

MUSCLE MASS

Do you remember in Chapter 3 when I told you I had spent some time on bed rest? Well, it turns out that when you lie on your back for almost two months, the body goes through some changes. For me, one of those was muscle atrophy. During my hospital stay, my legs shriveled to what can only be described as toothpicks.

Those legs were unrecognizable and no longer able to accommodate the weight of my slender frame. "How could this be?" I thought. I mean, I didn't do anything else but lie there while trying to bake a baby. Next thing I knew, my legs seemed to have wasted away.

Somewhere in our culture, it has been normalized and somewhat internalized that women don't need to weight train or maintain and build muscles. While my example of being on hospital bed rest is an extreme case, it's not too much to grasp that without intentional and consistent use, your muscles will waste away. Women especially have been overrun with the idea that weight training is for men, and all you need to do is run on a treadmill and look cute while doing it. While there have been some consistent strides in recent years to debunk this messaging, I found it important to address it here.

Muscle Loss, Bone Loss, and Aging

When it comes to aging and keeping a strong, healthy body, the prevention of osteoporosis is often one of the first considerations that come to mind. But age-related muscle loss, or sarcopenia, is also an unfortunate yet expected part of aging. By the time you're between the ages of thirty and thirty-five, you can expect to lose between 1 percent and 2 percent of muscle mass per year of life. After age sixty, that number jumps to 3 percent of muscle loss per year. In people older than seventy-five, that percentage is even higher. Ultimately, that boils down to four to six pounds of muscle loss every ten years.

Fragility due to sarcopenia is the main culprit for which more than three million seniors are treated in emergency rooms for serious fall injuries every year. The worst part is that these injuries are largely preventable. That's muscle that you just can't afford to lose. Walking is great and does build some muscle, but by itself it doesn't build the kind of muscle you need to fight sarcopenia.

The good news is that muscle loss doesn't have to accompany aging. You don't need a whole lot of time to start building muscle and start getting stronger. High-intensity resistance training just two to three times per week is enough to deter sarcopenia.

Not only will you increase strength, but weight-bearing exercises also increase bone density while decreasing the chances of osteoporosis. Exercises that use body weight such as push-ups, planks, and pull-ups all contribute to muscle tone and strength. If you're tight on space and want to get the benefits of adding weights to your exercise routine, you could also try using things such as ankle weights and resistance bands.

BEST TIME TO EXERCISE

Know Your Chronotype

Your chronotype is the inner wiring that determines how energetic or tired you are at what time of day. It's based on your circadian rhythm. Are you buzzing with energy at 6:00 in the morning, or are you in a semi-comatose state despite having adequate rest? Are you ready to turn in at 10:00 p.m., or is that when the party's just beginning? Most people refer to this as being a "morning person" or a "night owl," but there's a little more to it than that. While chronotype is greatly affected by genetics, other things such as exposure to sunlight, geographic location, age, and when you exercise can also have an impact.

Doctors and researchers have various ways to describe this, but according to Dr. Michael Breus, a fellow of the American Academy of Sleep Medicine, there are four main chronotypes.

Lion: This is a typical early bird persona—wide-eyed and bushy-tailed in the morning, and would opt for a morning matinee over an evening movie any day. If you fall into this category, your most productive time of day is before noon.

Bear: Most people fall into the bear chronotype category. This chronotype is considered intermediate between the extremes. If that's you, then you tend to be more productive or energetic a little later in the day, around noon. Your sleepfulness or wakefulness tends to follow the pattern of the sun.

Wolf: A wolf chronotype is more energetic later in the day and tends to want to sleep in. This is definitely not the person to call to join you for an early morning run. Someone with this chronotype gets additional waves of energy in the evening.

Dolphin: A smaller portion of the population has the dolphin chronotype. These individuals have a hard time finding a sleep schedule that works for them and often have insomnia. In spite of that, many find success exercising between 10:00 a.m. and 2:00 p.m.

What's the point? You can hack your productivity if you know your chronotype. You are also more likely to be successful sticking to an exercise routine if you take your chronotype into consideration. Why would you set your alarm clock to work out at 4:00 a.m. every day if you're clearly a wolf and that's your least productive time of day? Doesn't make sense, right?

A PUBLIC APOLOGY

This is the point in the book where I want to pause and apologize to all my late-night study group partners from my undergrad years and beyond. I tried desperately to pull late-nighters and all-nighters with you when biologically it was not my peak time of productivity. If only I had known then what I know now. I was studying with wolves when I'm all lion.

Own your biology! Own your life!

The More You Know, the More You Glow!

Although you should take your chronotype into consideration when choosing a time to exercise, take note that those who exercise between

8:00 a.m. and 11:00 a.m. have a lower risk of coronary heart disease. On the other hand, people who routinely exercise between 7:00 p.m. and 11:00 p.m. alter their circadian rhythm, which can disrupt beneficial sleep. The time of day you select is not just crucial from an energy perspective; it can affect your circadian rhythm.

DON'T FIND THE TIME - MAKE THE TIME

Another movement motivator that can help you work out more consistently is creating a consistent schedule and sticking to it.

Why is that important? Think about it this way: Most people would never dream of making a doctor's appointment and intentionally missing it. You may take time off from work, block off your schedule, put the appointment on all your calendars, and make sure you leave your house or office early enough so you don't get stuck in traffic. You would do everything in your power to avoid a late fee or miss the appointment entirely. After all, this is your health we're talking about. That "wellness" visit is important. The doctor's time is important.

The point is that every time you make time to work out, you're having your own wellness visit. Not only is your doctor's time important, but your time is important too. Wellness visits happen every time you take the stairs instead of the elevator, every time you choose water instead of juice, every time you spend thirty minutes doing cardio instead of plopping down and binge-watching your favorite show.

Wellness visits don't happen once a year; they happen *every day*.

DRESS TO IMPRESS

Dress to impress is not about impressing other people with what you're wearing to work out. Dress to impress is about impressing on yourself the importance of what you're doing. Working out is so important that you should outfit yourself with clothing that won't hinder your movement and makes you feel good.

You should wear shoes that enhance not hinder your stride, and reevaluate them often. Wear workout clothes that support how you *want* to feel forever versus how you may feel at the moment.

This matters whether you're working out at home or getting your movement on at a fancy sports club. Don't dare put on that workout video while you're still wearing your pajamas! Fabrics, colors, fit, and design matter. Seeing words of encouragement also matters. That is true whether those words are on your clothes or on the walls and environment around you.

These movement motivators are simple and efficient ways that can support your body's quest to sweat, move, and heal. Be good to your body so your body can be good to you.

MY TOP BELLY BULGE BUSTERS (BBB)

Let me start out by saying that you can't spot-reduce fat. This is not a magic show, and I'm not David Copperfield.

But over the years, I've spoken with enough people to know that this topic is a hot button across genders. Assuming you're already engaging in moderate to high-intensity aerobic activity a minimum of three times a week, here are my top belly bulge busters (BBBs).

(P.S. Yes, these BBBs will also work if you're peri- or postmenopausal.)

One of the keys to reducing belly fat is lowering blood insulin levels. Consistent high insulin levels cause the body to hold on to fat along the belly and waistline. Now that you know that, these BBBs will make even more sense.

Grain-free diet: That includes removing wheat and wheat products. Where do you think the term "beer belly" came from?

Intermittent fasting or time-restricted eating (TRE): This makes you metabolically fit and turns your body into a fat-burning machine.

No mindless snacking: You don't need a sweet treat after every meal.

Plank exercises: Keeps the core tight!

Limited alcoholic beverages! No elaboration needed.

Green tea: Green tea consumption is associated with weight control and an increase in metabolic activity.

Reduced sugar intake: Persistent consumption of HFCS, sugary drinks, cakes, cookies, sugar-laced gourmet coffees, and breads are enablers of belly bulge.

Increased muscle mass: Muscles use the majority of glucose in the blood. So the more muscles you have, the more controlled your blood sugar will be. The more controlled your blood sugar is, the fewer insulin spikes and the less belly fat you'll have.

DR. LISA'S NOTES

» You don't have to enjoy exercising to get motivated to move. There are six mindful movement motivators that can help keep you inspired to stay active.
» Use your chronotype to your advantage to determine the best time to exercise.

WELLNESS PRESCRIPTION

» Take a few minutes to determine your chronotype. You can use the descriptions in this chapter, and there are also fun quizzes you can access online to help guide you on the right path.

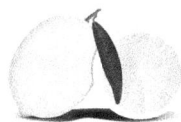

Chapter 25

ENERGY DRAINERS

Guard your energy like you guard your passwords.

If you or anyone you know has taken science classes, you probably already know the first law of thermodynamics—"Energy cannot be created or destroyed, only transformed from one form to another."

Our energy is one of the most valuable things we own. I often wonder why we give it away so freely.

Foods, activities, behaviors, environments, and people all fall into one of two categories: energy depleters and energy enhancers. We're going to cover both categories in this chapter and the next chapter.

Lack of energy, or fatigue, is one of the most common complaints people have. It's often said that if anyone knew how to bottle up the boatloads of energy of a small child and sell it, that business would be an immediate success.

When it comes to individual energy levels, *output* is determined by *input*. What you eat (or don't eat), your activity level, and your nutrition are key. But most people don't want to hear the basics. Everyone is looking for that magic pill or magic "juice" to get the energy they need. The problem is that millions of people have been zapped clean.

To illustrate this, just look at the growth of the coffee industry. In the United States alone, the revenue from coffee has been valued at $80 billion. And while some people are after flavor and aroma in a cup of their favorite brew, let's face it, for many, the best part of waking up is a little jolt of energy in your cup.

Since I've already written extensively about food, nutrition, and exercise, this chapter will focus on other ignored aspects of energy generation and energy depletion—your surrounding environment and rest.

Your body is like a cell phone. At times it's fully charged, and at other times it's near depletion and needs recharging. Think about your phone for a moment. You probably have it near you right now. What kind of things quickly deplete your phone's battery?

I'm not your phone service company, but I can tell you that things like running too many apps and programs in the background, streaming video, recording video, picture taking, leaving the phone in the sun, always having the phone on, and using the phone display at maximum brightness are all things that quickly deplete a phone's battery. I'm sure you can think of some other things to put on the list.

Just as there are things that can drain your phone's battery, there are things you do (knowingly or unknowingly) that deplete your energy.

Remember, you picked up this book to lean into the uncomfortable so you will be more amiable to change. It's this change that can and will transform your health and your life for the better.

That being said, let's talk about some energy drainers in your environment (besides food) that could be negatively affecting your battery life and how you can change them.

TOP 8 ENERGY DEPLETERS

Here are my top eight energy depleters. How many of them affect you?

1. Working in a Job or Industry You Hate

Being in a job or industry you hate or no longer believe in will drain your energy like no other.

Trust me, I know.

When you consider that a whopping one-third of life is spent at work, having a mismatch of interests, industry, or environment can wreak havoc on your health.

It's interesting how people spend so much time preaching to their kids that "you can be anything you want to be," but somehow they think those words don't apply to them or their stage in life.

The issue is that in today's society, we place more value on money and prestige than on natural passion, talents, and interests.

If you're interested in exploring this topic more, the resources below can help you start to transition toward working in alignment with your strengths and not against them. Here are some tools to help get you there.

- Clifton Strengthsfinder
- Kolbe Test
- VIA Character and Strength Survey and Character Report

2. Toxic Relationships (Intimate, Familial, Friendships, or Other)

It doesn't matter what type of relationship you're in. Consistent negativity or strain has no place in your Be FINE life. Heal the relationships that need to heal, redefine boundaries for ones you're going to keep, and let go of those you need to let go of. That's it.

There are two types of people in your life—energy drainers and energy enhancers. Analyze your squad, and adjust accordingly.

3. Energy-Draining Food

I'm not going to hammer this one over your head since we already did that in the food part of this book. But anything that is overly processed, non-organic, dye-filled, or genetically modified is considered energy-draining food. And if that food causes inflammation in your body, you'd better cut it out, or it will cut you down. If you have more questions on what these foods are, refer back to the "F" in FINE.

4. Electromagnetic Fields (EMF)

You may not think of it this way, but humans are electrical beings. Certain things charge you up, and others drain your battery. Electric signals are generated in the brain and travel to other parts of the body to think, move, process, and even heal. The body does that through the original information superhighway—the nervous system.

In today's modern world, there's an onslaught of human-made electromagnetic fields (EMFs) that are always present and act as energy drainers.

While there are both natural (from the earth) and human-made EMFs, the latter is what is of concern.

Human-made EMFs come from manufactured electric sources. The energy is transmitted through the use of electrical equipment such as component wiring, mobile phones, smart devices, and electrical transformers.

EMFs are used in many contexts, including powering residential security systems, heating up leftover dinners, listening to your favorite podcast, and catching up with a friend on your cell phone. While technology is certainly useful, it's your responsibility to learn how to use that technology wisely. Don't expect the manufacturers of the products that emit EMFs to tell you how to do it.

The present-day barrage of human-made EMFs is a source of electromagnetic pollution and has been implicated in a myriad of harmful effects, from stress to sleep disturbances and even harmful chronic conditions. One study showed that electromagnetic radiation produced by cell phones can produce tumors in lab animals.

Even so, some entities continue to say that more research is needed in this area and state that current health findings are inconclusive. Despite this, toxicology studies point to some serious health consequences that cannot be ignored. As a result, every attempt should be made to limit EMF exposure whenever possible.

What You Don't Know Can Hurt You

I knew someone who was suffering with insomnia for years. She told me that she had been to the best sleep doctors and even took part in a sleep study, but no one could get to the bottom of her condition. I asked her if she would be open to trying a very simple solution she could use that night that would not cost her anything.

She was very dubious but ultimately agreed.

Do you want to know what the tip was?

I told her, "Tonight before you go to sleep, put your phone on airplane mode, and turn off the Wi-Fi in your home."

(Before you start freaking out, continue reading. In the next section, I'll list some alternative options for people who want to stay plugged in.)

The next day, she called me, screaming ecstatically, "You're a genius. Oh my gosh! You're a genius! Last night I slept like a baby for the first time in years!"

While I can't say that her experience will be yours, it's worth learning from.

The thing is, I'm not a genius. I just know that the human body is an electromagnetic force that can't be ignored or denied. Applying electromagnetic energy to the body from any source will positively or negatively affect the human experience.

It doesn't matter if you can see it or not. It doesn't matter how many big tech companies say their products are safe. It doesn't even matter if you believe it or not. What matters is how your body interprets those electromagnetic fields.

So here are some simple things you can do to take charge of the energy in your space.

- Put your phone on airplane mode before you go to bed. And even better, leave it outside your bedroom.
- Put your computer on airplane mode when it's not in use.
- Use an analog or manual clock as your alarm clock.
- Avoid putting internet routers in your bedroom.
- Turn off your Wi-Fi at night, or use an EMF cage.

Wi-Fi routers are one of the biggest culprits of electromagnetic pollution in the home. If you aren't able to disconnect your Wi-Fi before bed due to security camera usage, computer use, or other variables, consider buying a Faraday box or EMF cage to put your router in. Using one of them reduces exposure to radiation but still allows you to jump on the internet at a moment's notice.

You can also get a separate Faraday bag for your cell phone, or put the phone in another room at night. One of the worst things you can do is sleep with the phone by your head, in your bed, or on your body. And while I'm at it, if you're wearing your phone near your chest or pushing it into your bra before taking the dog for a walk or going for a run . . . please stop! I see you! You're literally guiding the EMF signals to your most precious organs while also putting delicate breast tissue in harm's way.

The point is to minimize EMF exposure whenever you can.

Besides minimizing electromagnetic pollution, one of the additional benefits of staying disconnected from your phone during bedtime is that when you wake up, you have more control of what receives your mental energy. This is a great way to avoid filling your head with intrusive notifications, unwanted emails, and news alerts first thing in the morning.

Instead, make time to tell God "hello," read from a devotional, your Bible, or other positive reading, and set your intentions for the day.

Like I mentioned, don't freak out.

I have an option if you need to be able to keep the line of communication open overnight.

For Those Still Freaking Out after I Actually Said "Don't Freak Out"

Whether you have kids, grown adults, grandkids, or just need to be available for a loved one or spouse, it's important to always have a lifeline available to those you love. No one wants the kind of call that comes at 3:00 in the morning. Yet still, especially when you have kids, you need to be available at all times in case of emergencies. If your phone is off or on airplane mode, you won't be able to get the call.

That's where landlines come in. Do you remember those? Having a hardwired phone available to those you love will allow communication in times of emergencies while still allowing for reduced EMF exposure. It's a win-win.

Sleep is a very restorative process, so it's very important to reduce EMFs in your home, especially at bedtime.

Okay, that was a lot. But when you *know* better, you can *do* better. So here's your chance.

Do better.

5. Scaryvision

Fear sells. Fear is also an immunosuppressant, which means it suppresses the immune system.

One of the biggest producers of fear is sitting right in your family room. Perhaps there is also one sitting in your bedroom. Maybe another is sitting in the kitchen, and if you've really succeeded at "modernizing" your home, you may have one in your basement or media center.

It's your television screen.

It's not that TVs are inherently bad; it's that the programming we allow ourselves to be exposed to in the name of keeping informed and entertained is not always "good news."

I'm not here to tell you what to watch, but be mindful of the energy you allow into your personal space.

If you're constantly in a state of fear, you won't have to go and find illness; it will easily come and find you.

6. Social Media

Like TV, social media is not inherently evil. As a digital content creator, online publisher, and virtual shop owner, I've worked in social media for well over a decade. It has allowed me to do some wonderful things such as being on national and local TV shows, taking my family on a once-in-a-lifetime vacation, meeting some amazing people, landing my own online series, connecting with estranged family, getting access to amazing products, and building an online platform where I get to help people from all over the world.

The problem is not social media. The problem is how it's used and how often it's used. Let's talk about some strategic digital wellness tips on how to use social media more healthfully.

I'm sorry, but I won't be able to tell you who to "friend," what to share, or who should be in your "close friends circle." However, these quick tips will help you establish some healthy boundaries so social media is less of an energy depleter in your life.

It really just comes down to a few things.

Turn off push notifications. Push notifications are a way to keep you coming back to apps and social media sites. They don't care if you are in the middle of exercise, reading your child a bedtime story, or in the middle listening to one of your friends' never-ending stories. The more you keep coming back to the app, the more ads you'll see, and the more money they'll make.

At the end of the day, social media apps are businesses and not your wellness coach. So do yourself a favor, and keep push notifications off.

Set up electronic downtime and limits. You may not know this, but in your phone's settings, you can set up downtimes and specific app limits to improve digital wellness. You can set limits per social media app or for your phone as a whole. Don't worry. You'll be able to use your phone during this time for other things such as making phone calls. This simple step puts you in charge of social media so social media is not in charge of you.

Another technique that works well for some people is removing social media apps on their phone altogether and just using them on a laptop or desktop.

Take wellness weekends. If you're having difficulty limiting social media, wellness weekends are another way to put yourself back in the driver's seat. Although weekends officially include Saturdays and Sundays, I recommend starting your wellness weekend anytime between Friday afternoon or evening and ending it on Sunday evening or Monday morning.

It's just a few days off, but it can make a big difference in terms of maintaining a positive mental mindset. It's your wellness weekend. Adjust the schedule as you see fit to get the most out of it.

7. Blue Light

You may be reading this and wondering what a blue light is and what the problem is with it? First, it's not all blue light that is the problem—it's *artificial* blue light.

Blue light is a type of EMF made of short wavelengths of high-energy light. Natural blue light comes from the sun as part of its white light. Artificial blue light comes from LED lamps, mobile phones, computers, tablets, fluorescent lights, e-readers, TVs, and more.

Natural blue light has to travel a long distance before it gets to earth, so it's not as much of a concern. In addition, most people don't spend nearly as much time in the sun as they do using and watching electrical devices. The average American now spends more than eleven hours in front of screens every day.

That's almost half a day!

While exposure to natural blue light from the sun helps set circadian rhythm to improve alertness, blue light from artificial light sources such as lamps, smart screens, televisions, phones, and computers have the opposite effect.

The problem with artificial blue light is that it's a recent modern phenomenon with damaging consequences that likely didn't exist when your parents were growing up. Exposure to artificial blue light at night can cause digital eye strain, headaches, and disturbances in sleep. It's always baffling to me the number of people who post on social media at 2:00 or 3:00 in the morning and then complain about having a hard time falling asleep. The irony of this situation is that the very thing they are using for comfort is likely the cause of the insomnia that plagues them.

To help you get around this, here are some things you can do to limit exposure to blue light at night. On your mobile phone, go into settings and then to display settings, and turn on night vision. It may be called a different name, depending on what type of phone you have and when you're reading this.

For example, on my phone this setting is called "night vision." On my friend's phone, it's called "eye comfort shield."

Turning on this setting will allow your phone to use darker screen colors at night while lowering blue light emittance, decreasing the chances of eye damage, and allowing you to get a more restful night's sleep. Remember, this setting is not automatically turned on. You have to look for it and turn it on yourself to reap the benefits.

When it comes to computer use, most modern computers have a setting you can turn on for decreased blue light exposure at night. Typically, you can alter this setting based on your location or do it manually—whatever suits you best.

When it comes to reducing the blue light from TV screens, you have a few options. The easiest option is to wear a good pair of blue-light-blocking glasses when you watch TV at night. Another option is to invest in a blue light TV screen protector.

If none of these options suit you, remember that turning off the TV is a viable option!

8. Personal Pollutants

I'm not going to go all EPA on you. I'm just not the one. But if we're going to talk about energy drainers in your environment, we have to discuss personal pollutants. The goal is to limit the number of chemicals in your home. If you care about your health, continue reading to find out how.

Bisphenols are one of the biggest threats when it comes to maintaining personal well-being. These additives comprise of a group of chemicals used in the manufacturing of plastics. To combat the negative health effects, one of the most beneficial things you can do is limit the use of plastic when storing or heating food.

Research has shown that chemicals used in plastics—bisphenol A (BPA), bisphenol B (BPB), and bisphenol S (BPS)—can find their way into food and cause negative health effects. Potential side effects include hormone disruption, increased cancer risk, and altered behavior, especially in young kids.

While you may think you're in the clear because you use products labeled "BPA free," its close cousins BPB and BPS are no better. Obviously, none of us can avoid all toxin exposure, but even small lifestyle changes can make a big difference.

Since I know you're already eager to make some changes by buying organic non-GMO food, you might as well go ahead and buy the right containers to store the food in.

Instead of storing food in plastic containers, a healthier alternative is glass, porcelain, or stainless steel containers. That is especially true when heating up food. Heating food in plastic containers makes it more likely that those chemicals will leach into the food and be ingested.

OUTDOOR AIR IS CLEANER THAN INDOOR AIR

The truth shall set you free. And the truth is that the air outside your home is often cleaner than the air inside your home. You can go ahead and thank the prevalence of indoor pollutants for that one.

To decrease the amount of indoor pollutants circulating in your home or office space, there are a few things you can do right now that will help.

How to Decrease Indoor Air Pollution in Your Home

- Invest in a few quality air purifiers with high-efficiency particulate air filtration (HEPA) filters.
- Make sure to change air filters according to the manufacturer's instructions.
- When cooking, turn on the vent hood to get rid of cooking odors and accumulating air contaminants.
- Open doors and windows during warm weather months to get fresh air circulating inside.
- Limit wearing outdoor shoes in indoor spaces. Like they do in Japan, remove your outdoor shoes at the door, and put on your indoor slippers.
- Vacuum carpeted and high traffic areas frequently.

All these things will help to clear the air and support your body on your journey to being well.

DR. LISA'S NOTES

» You are responsible for your energy. Guard it well!
» Foods, activities, behaviors, environments, and people fall into one of two categories: Energy depleters and energy enhancers. Determine which one you're dealing with, and adjust accordingly.
» Energy depleters are all around you! Learn how to control them, or they will control you.

WELLNESS PRESCRIPTION

» Inspect your home for sources of EMF and blue light that may be acting as energy depleters on your body.
» Next, come up with two solutions you can implement this week to limit their use or reduce their EMF impact.

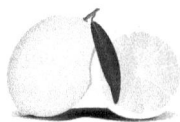

Chapter 26

ENERGY ENHANCERS

*If you don't take care of your body, how do
you expect it to take care of you?*

In the previous chapter, we talked about the various things that can
deplete your human battery. Many of these energy depleters fly under
the radar unnoticed. That's why I devoted a lot of time to them.

Similar to a cell phone battery, you are affected by various energy
depleters and energy enhancers in your life. They can either enhance
your battery power or deplete it.

Let's look at that cell phone example. You occasionally have to turn off
the phone and plug it in to recharge the battery. That is one of the best
things you can do to recharge the phone in order to optimize battery life.

Fortunately, when it comes to the human body, there are many energy
enhancers you can take advantage of. Most of them were covered in previous parts of this book. Some examples include organic non-GMO fruits
and vegetables, non-inflammatory foods, intermittent fasting, immunity
boosters, positive mindset, exercise, and proper elimination.

Still, there is one big energy enhancer we haven't covered yet. One
of the best ways for the body to increase energy, improve longevity, and
enhance performance is to power off everything and recharge through
adequate, quality sleep.

THE JOYS OF SLEEP!

I recently asked this question in my private online community: "When was the last time you had a good night's sleep?"

The first response was this: "Ten years ago!"

The answer is funny, but then it's not.

Lack of quality sleep is no laughing matter. In fact, sleep deprivation is one of the biggest reasons people are walking around chronically fatigued. As many as 70 million Americans are currently affected by some type of sleep-related problem. Health consequences of sleep-related disorders and lack of quality sleep include sleep apnea, hypertension, diabetes, stroke, cognitive decline, chronic fatigue, and the inability to resist diseases and infections such as the common cold.

The truth is, we live in an "every day I'm hustlin, I'll sleep when I'm dead" kind of world. But sleep is not as disposable as society would have you believe. Sure, no one gets through the newborn baby phase unscathed, but getting adequate sleep is a vital part of proper health and well-being.

Lack of quality sleep is associated with unwanted weight gain. Specifically, sleep deprivation affects hormones such as ghrelin and leptin. Ghrelin is an appetite-stimulating hormone that lowers the level of hunger satisfaction. Leptin is a hormone that acts as an appetite suppressant. The loss of just one night of sleep per week is enough to increase ghrelin and decrease leptin. You eat more, fostering unwanted weight gain.

Decreased sleep also causes an increase in cortisol, a stress hormone. The prolonged release of cortisol can promote the storage of belly fat and affect the metabolism of carbohydrates, leading to high blood sugar.

Increased cortisol release can also cause elevated oil production, leading to clogged pores and breakouts. Now you know the reason they call it beauty sleep!

Quality sleep promotes cell and body renewal, as well as restoration. Some of the restorative processes that happen during sleep include protein synthesis, the release of hormones, tissue growth, muscle synthesis, and waste removal.

If you're looking for fewer wrinkles, smoother skin, clearer thoughts, more energy, tissue repair, and increased immunity, spend some time getting quality sleep. Those light cat naps are just not going to cut it. Rest and restoration is so important that even God rested on the seventh day. The bottom line is that sleep is not disposable.

Dr. Lisa's Sleep Tips

To help you get the quality sleep you need, here are some tips on how to get a better night's rest, starting tonight.

Keep the Temperature Low

It's been shown that the best temperature for sleep is around 65°F. As a result, many sleep professionals recommend keeping the thermostat between 60 and 67°F at bedtime. If you're having temperature wars with your partner, say that you're just doing the best thing for your health, and that should help you win the battle.

Turn Off the Wi-Fi or Use a Protective Cage

For reasons mentioned in Chapter 25, turn off the Wi-Fi or get an EMF cage to cover your router at night. Put your cell phone on airplane mode or in a separate room at bedtime. You can use a manual alarm clock to keep things on schedule. As a best practice, do not store the phone in your bed or near your body, especially at night.

Establish a Bedtime Routine

One of the great things about being an adult is going to bed at any time you want.

One of the irresponsible things about being an adult is going to bed at any time you want.

Establish a bedtime routine that includes a shower or bath, the use of relaxing essential oils such as lavender and ylang ylang, and a relaxing read or journal entry before bed. Go to bed at a reasonable hour according to your chronotype. Most adults need at least eight hours of uninterrupted sleep-in order to feel rested and energetic the next morning.

Decrease Blue Light Exposure

Change the settings on your phone, computer, and other electronic devices to decrease blue light exposure. Blue light disrupts your circadian rhythm and the body's ability to regenerate hormones. Stop using electronics at least one hour before bedtime.

Hold the Caffeine

For a positive and restorative sleep experience, avoid caffeine at least six hours before bedtime since it has been shown to cause disruptive sleep.

In addition, caffeine is a diuretic. Drinking caffeinated drinks too close to bedtime can cause excessive urination. Waking up to use the bathroom is the definition of disruptive sleep. Avoid it if you can.

Midnight Snacks

Whoever came up with the idea of midnight snacking obviously didn't understand the importance of establishing good sleep hygiene. To avoid heartburn, gastric upset, slowed metabolism, and waking up in the middle of the night to use the bathroom, avoid eating meals and snacks at least three hours before bedtime.

DR. LISA'S NOTES

» One of the biggest energy enhancers is sleep.
» Sleep deprivation can cause a myriad of health problems, including hypertension, stroke, uncontrolled weight gain, skin eruptions, and increased risk of infection and disease.

WELLNESS PRESCRIPTION

» Set a bedtime for yourself this week, and stick to it.
» For better sleep, use at least three of the tips listed above, and then dedicate a solid eight hours for sleep tonight. Take notice of how great you feel the next day!

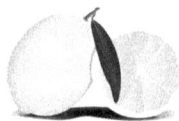

Chapter 27

BECOME YOUR FINE SELF!

There are two secrets to better health: Start, and don't stop.

Oh my goodness! You did it! You really did it!

You should feel proud of yourself for making it to the last chapter of this book. As a matter of fact, stop whatever you're doing right now
    and give yourself a standing ovation.

I promise, it's not weird or anything. You deserve this.

That was the easy part.

The next step is to use this book as a guide and trusted resource for empowered health for the rest of your life.

And guess what?

To do this you're going to have to read this book again!

This time, take notes.

Highlight the parts that grab you.

Reread some choice bits, and try and try again.

And above all, never give up on yourself.

When it comes down to it, there are two secrets to better health.

The first secret is to start.

The second is to never stop.

Your health and your life are way too important to ever surrender!

When it comes to personal health, there are always signs when things are moving in the wrong direction. Similar to the presence of tremors before a big earthquake, stop and think, "What are the tremors in your life?"

Is it tingling in your hands and feet? Do you get recurrent yeast infections or fibroids? Do you suffer from migraines? Memory lapses? Are there uncontrolled weight fluctuations or sleep disruptions? Are there aches and pains? Is your hair thinning or falling out?

Don't wait for a big earthquake before you figure things out.

When it comes down to it, what you value most always comes to the surface. And let's be honest, it's not that you don't have time. It's that you won't *make time* for what matters most.

YOU!

Taking care of everyone else but yourself is not selfless! It's *self-harm*. The only way to counter that harm is to put yourself at the top of the list.

Banish the excuses.

Build appropriate boundaries.

Bridge the gap.

Learn how to take charge of your health from the inside out, not the outside in.

Your body requires deliberate action to facilitate the restoration of wellness.

When I was growing up, it was a great compliment when someone said, "You look fine." It meant I looked better than good.

It had nothing to do with how I felt, how healthy I was, or the likelihood that I would live a long and independent life.

I get it. You want what's on the outside to look good, but what's happening on the *inside* is so much more important. Whether or not I've always recognized it as such, wellness has always been a part of my mission and my passion. Through the years, I've seen health trends and fads come and go. But the truth is that wellness is not a fad. It's a way of life.

It's based on key principles that have stood the test of time. The more recent challenge has been navigating those key principles in our modern world where there is a pill for every ill and using natural modalities to heal is quieted versus amplified.

I've always felt like there needed to be a health and wellness book that was comprehensive yet written with a relatable "I'm your friend next door" tone. After seeing so many around me struggle in the battle for their lives, I realized that I needed to do something more. I needed to write the book I wanted to read.

I hope you learn from this book, grow from it, get healthier, and free yourself from the medical chains of sickcare that may be holding you back. It's often said that it takes an average of 17 years for scientific research to reach clinical practice. That number doesn't even account for the fact that there is tremendous bias in what type of studies get researched.

The point? If you're waiting for a landmark study that demonstrates a decreased prevalence of cancer risk based on increased serum vitamin D levels and then waiting for your physician to put that recommendation into clinical practice, you'll be better off expecting a golden egg from a goose.

Anyway, enough with the nursery rhymes. It was challenging to get paragraphs of this book written between homeschool lessons, travel, and the crazy balance of an entrepreneurial family, but alas, we've come to the end of the book.

Actually, it's the beginning of your journey to better health.

I can still hear my nine-year-old son incredulously asking, "You're not finished with that book yet?"

And my twelve-year-old daughter assuredly asked, "Once you're done, I can read the book for free, right?"

What can I say? They help keep me accountable.

Now it's your turn. It's your turn to be accountable to yourself. In this book, you have discovered how to nourish to flourish, decrease inflammation, increase immunity, optimize nutrients, and eliminate the junk in order to have more energy and vitality than you've ever known. Be FINE is the drug-free playbook to age well, beat bulge, and stop disease—what you've always needed but couldn't find.

Now that you have it, the question is, what are you going to do with it?

My guess is that you'll Be FINE:

Focus, Fiber, Fuel
Inflammation and Immunity
Nutrition
Elimination, Exercise, Energy

Now go on with your **FINE** self!

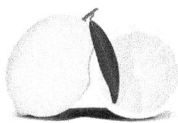

Chapter 28

YOUR FINE NUTRITION PLAN

Change your food, change your life.

You're finished with the book. Now what? I can hear you asking, "So, what am I going to eat?"

Don't worry. I won't leave you hanging.

As Benjamin Franklin said, "If you fail to plan, you are planning to fail!" Remember, some foods are life-givers while others are life-stealers.

It's just that simple.

As a wellness warrior, I want to see you not just survive but *thrive*. You are on a crazy cycle of life, and the bottom line is that your nutritional needs are not getting met. So I've prepared a FINE plan just for you.

Consider it your lifeline. In this chapter and the next are more than two weeks of meal ideas, a sample meal plan, and more than enough recipes to get you started on your wellness journey.

LET'S GET STARTED!

Food is an integral part of living and being well. As such, I've included some of my favorite mouth-watering recipes to try. These recipes were intuitively and nutritionally crafted to help you attain better health, attenuate dietary deficiencies, minimize disease, optimize well-being—and taste delicious!

The recipes are full of fresh ingredients, tantalizing spices, and satisfying herbs. My special FINE plan will allow you to take better control of your health and your life one tasty bite at a time.

A Note about Ingredients

These recipes should be prepared using organic, non-GMO ingredients, pasture-raised chicken and eggs, grass-fed and grass-finished beef, and wild-sourced seafood when possible.

"That sounds expensive," you might reply.

Consider this. It's less expensive than the cost of sick days, excessive doctors' visits, unnecessary surgeries, painful procedures, and potentially toxic medications.

It's Good Fat

When cooking, extra virgin olive oil, avocado oil, and ghee are preferred. Coconut oil can also be used, but it's not neutral in flavor.

Ghee is made from butter that has been cooked on low heat until all the milk solids have been removed. That includes removal of casein and lactose. As a result, ghee is a good choice for those who are dairy-sensitive. After cooking the butter and removing the milk solids, the end product is smooth, creamy, and filled with anti-inflammatory and therapeutic benefits.

Choose a brand made from grass-fed, pasture-raised cows. It has a high smoke point, which is ideal for cooking. Ghee is known to increase the absorption and nutritional value of herbs and is used in Ayurvedic medicine.

If you can't get your hands on ghee, you can use butter made from grass-fed, grass-finished cows.

All Salt Is Not Created Equal

For the purposes of meal preparation, all salt should be natural and unrefined. Examples include Himalayan salt, Real Salt, and Celtic salt and other ancient salts.

MEAL IDEAS

Break the Fast	Soups, Salads, Sides, & Sips	Main Dishes
Almond flour banana pancakes	Butternut squash apple bisque	Baked salmon balls
Coconut chia pudding	Callaloo-style greens	Beanless chili
Creamy almond porridge	Chesapeake shrimp salad	Caribbean shrimp creole
Crunchy grain-free granola	Cilantro cauliflower rice	Coconut curry shrimp
Flaxseed quinoa porridge	Crispy sweet potato rounds	Coconut-lime chicken
Grain-free carrot muffins	Cucumber salad	Grilled (soy-free) teriyaki salmon
Green lean scramble	Curry chicken salad	Honey ginger shrimp
Perfect soft or hard-boiled eggs	Easy egg salad	Island-style curry chicken
Pina colada smoothie bowl	Green onion herb sauce	Kale and mushroom frittata
	Green pea skin-brightening smoothie	Lemon herb chicken
	Honey ginger beer	Mexican style chicken skewers
	Kale mashed potatoes	Pesto chicken
	Mango blueberry salad	Spicy beef stew
	Mashed green bananas	
	Roasted carrots and green beans	
	Sauteed lemon kale	
	Sisserou chicken quinoa salad	
	Stew papaya	
	Slim ting Virgin Islands potato stuffing	
	Trafalgar tropical smoothie	
	Warm Dijon potato salad with caramelized onions	

SAMPLE ANTI-INFLAMMATORY MEAL PLAN

First Meal	Second Meal	Third Meal
Almond flour banana pancakes, boiled eggs, broccoli sprouts	Mango blueberry salad (add leftover grilled chicken breasts or other protein of choice)	Curried chicken, callaloo style greens, stewed papaya
Cauliflower rice power bowl: cilantro lime cauliflower rice, smoked salmon, fried eggs, diced tomatoes, diced avocados, green onion herb sauce	Baked salmon balls, baked sweet potato, sauteed lemon kale	Caribbean shrimp creole, cilantro lime cauliflower rice, steamed broccoli
Creamy almond porridge topped with blueberries and walnuts	Curry chicken salad on a bed of greens	Coconut-lime chicken, mashed green bananas, callaloo style greens
Green lean scramble, sliced ripe avocados, green onion herb sauce	Sisserou chicken quinoa salad, side of arugula	Spicy beef stew, green salad
Flaxseed quinoa porridge	Easy egg salad on a bed of greens	Pesto chicken, warm Dijon potato salad, fresh broccoli sprouts

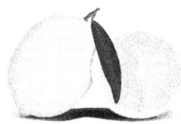

Chapter 29

RECIPES

ALMOND FLOUR BANANA PANCAKES

Serves: 6

Ingredients

1 cup blanched almond flour
1 cup tapioca flour
1 tsp baking powder
1/8 tsp salt
1 large egg (beaten)
2 bananas (mashed)
1 cup almond milk (unsweetened)
1/2 tsp vanilla extract
1 tbsp coconut oil (melted)
coconut oil spray for skillet or griddle
chopped raw walnuts
organic maple syrup

Directions

1. Preheat the skillet or griddle to medium high heat.
2. In a large bowl, mix dry ingredients (almond flour, tapioca flour, baking powder, and salt).
3. To the egg add the other wet ingredients (mashed bananas, almond milk, vanilla extract, melted coconut oil), mixing after each addition.
4. Add wet ingredients to dry ingredients. Do not overmix.
5. Grease the skillet lightly with coconut oil spray, wiping off any excess with a paper towel.
6. Use a ladle to place the batter on the preheated skillet.
7. Once bubbles start to appear on the batter, flip carefully. Cook for a few minutes before removing from heat.
8. Keep the pan lightly oiled between batches.
9. Serve with chopped walnuts and maple syrup as desired.

BAKED SALMON BALLS WITH ORANGE PINEAPPLE DIPPING SAUCE

Serves 4 (12 balls)

Ingredients

(Salmon Balls)

2 cans (6 oz) wild canned salmon (drained)
Juice of 1/2 lemon
1/3 cup red pepper (chopped)
1/2 tsp fresh cracked black pepper
1 tbsp scallion, chopped (white and green)
1/2 tbsp Worcestershire sauce
1 tsp seafood seasoning of your choice
3 tbsp mayonnaise
1 cup almond flour (finely ground) divided into two equal parts
Coconut oil spray

(Orange Pineapple Dipping Sauce)

3/4 cup orange juice
1/2 cup pineapple juice
3 tbsp raw honey
1 clove garlic (minced)
1 tbsp ginger (finely chopped)
1/4 tsp crushed red pepper flakes

Directions

(Salmon Balls)

1. Preheat oven to 400°F.
2. Drain canned salmon, and put in a medium-sized bowl.
3. Mash and flake with a fork.
4. Add lemon juice, red pepper, black pepper, scallions, Worcestershire sauce, seafood seasoning, and mayonnaise.
5. Mix until thoroughly incorporated.
6. Add half the almond flour to the bowl, and continue to mix.
7. Scoop heaping tablespoons of the salmon mixture into your hands, and roll gently into balls.

8. Roll in remaining almond flour.
9. Place on a liberally oiled sheet pan.
10. Lightly spray tops of salmon balls with additional coconut oil spray, or drizzle with olive oil.
11. Bake for 20 minutes.
12. Broil on high for an additional 5 minutes.
13. Remove from the oven.
14. Serve with Orange Pineapple Dipping Sauce (below) or a dipping sauce of your choice.

(Orange Pineapple Dipping Sauce)

1. Place the ingredients for the dipping sauce in a small pot on medium heat.
2. Stir gently, and simmer for 15–20 minutes or until liquid begins to thicken.
3. Strain the liquid.
4. Drizzle over salmon balls or serve alongside for dipping.

BEANLESS CHILI

Serves 8–10

Ingredients

1 tbsp ghee
5 cloves (minced garlic)
1 large onion (diced)
8 oz stew beef
8 oz beef sirloin (cut in cubes)
1 cup beef broth
2 tsp sea salt
2 tbsp ground cumin
1 tsp all-purpose seasoning
1 tsp dry thyme
3 tbsp chili powder
2 (10 oz) cans diced tomatoes with green chili
2 (14 oz) cans tomato sauce
1 (4.5 oz) can tomato paste, about 1/2 cup
2 bay leaves
Garnishes: scallions, cilantro, sliced avocado

Directions

1. In ghee, saut the garlic and diced onion on low heat until soft and translucent (20–30 minutes).
2. Remove and set aside.
3. Brown stew beef and beef sirloin in small batches, and remove from the pan.
4. Add beef broth to the hot pan, using a wooden spoon to scrape up the tiny bits at the bottom before reserving the liquid.
5. Add browned beef and the beef broth to a slow cooker.
6. Add sautéed onions and garlic, salt, cumin, all-purpose seasoning, thyme, chili powder, diced tomatoes, tomato sauce, tomato paste, and bay leaves.
7. Cook in the slow cooker on high for 4 hours.
8. Remove bay leaves just before serving.
9. Garnish with scallions, cilantro, or sliced avocado as desired.

BUTTERNUT SQUASH APPLE BISQUE

Serves 4

Ingredients

1/2 yellow onion (sliced)
1 butternut squash (cut into rounds, 1 inch think)
2 tbsp olive oil
2 cups apple juice
1/2 tsp ground cumin
1/2 tsp cayenne pepper
1/2 tsp ground allspice
1/2 tsp cinnamon
2 bunches fresh thyme
1/2 tsp sea salt
1 tsp fresh cracked black pepper

Directions

1. Preheat oven to 400°F.
2. Line a heavy-duty baking pan with slices of fresh yellow onion.
3. Place slices of butternut squash over the onions to cover, so the onion slices are not exposed.
4. Brush tops of squash with olive oil, drizzling any remaining.
5. Bake 45 minutes or until tender.
6. Remove from the oven.
7. Use a spoon to carefully remove seeds from the centers of the cooked squash.
8. Next, remove the pulp from the skin, and discard the skin.
9. Place the butternut squash and the onions in a high-powered blender.
10. Add apple juice, herbs, spices, and seasonings (cumin, cayenne, allspice, cinnamon, thyme, salt, and pepper).
11. If your blender has a soup setting, use it to blend the soup.
12. Otherwise, blend all ingredients at high speed until creamy and smooth.
13. If your soup is cool after blending, reheat it on the stovetop on low for a few minutes.
14. Enjoy the delicious creaminess!

CALLALOO-STYLE GREENS

Serves 8–10

Ingredients

1 large bunch dark leafy greens (kale or collards will do)
2 cups water
1 tbsp olive oil
3 garlic cloves (minced)
1 small onion (sliced)
6 sprigs fresh thyme
10 oz frozen okra
10 oz cut frozen spinach
1 tsp apple cider vinegar
1/2 cup red pepper (diced)
1–2 tsp salt
1/2 tsp fresh ground pepper
1/2 tsp hot pepper sauce

Directions

1. Fill a large bowl with cold water.
2. Soak the collard greens in the water for 30 minutes. Make sure they are submerged.
3. Drain the water, and remove the hard stems and ribs.
4. Tear greens into bite-sized pieces.
5. Preheat a large pot on medium-low heat, and add olive oil.
6. Sauté garlic, onion, and thyme for a few minutes (be careful not to burn them).
7. Add collard greens, water, okra, spinach, apple cider vinegar, and red pepper.
8. Season with salt and pepper.
9. Stir to combine.
10. Cook covered for 30 minutes or until greens are tender.
11. Season with your favorite hot pepper sauce.

CARIBBEAN SHRIMP CREOLE

Serves 6

Ingredients

1 tbsp ghee
1 tbsp olive oil
1 medium yellow onion (chopped)
1/4 cup green onion (chopped)
3 cloves garlic (minced)
1 cup celery (chopped)
5 sprigs thyme
1/2 cup red pepper (chopped)
1/2 Scotch bonnet pepper (seeds removed)
1 cup water
2 tomatoes (diced)
1 tbsp tomato paste
1/2 tsp all-purpose seasoning
1/2 tsp paprika
1/2 tsp salt
1 whole bay leaf
1 lb medium-sized shrimp (peeled, shelled, and deveined)
Juice of 1/2 lime
1/4 cup fresh parsley (chopped)

Directions

1. Preheat a large skillet to medium heat.
2. Add ghee and olive oil.
3. Sauté onions (yellow and green), garlic, celery, thyme, and all peppers for about 5 minutes, until soft.
4. To the cup of water add tomatoes, tomato paste, all-purpose seasoning, paprika, salt, and bay leaf, and stir.
5. Simmer on low (mostly covered) for 25 minutes.
6. Add shrimp, and lime juice, and stir for a few minutes more.
7. Shrimp should curl and become opaque once cooked.
8. Scatter with chopped parsley the last 5 minutes of cooking.
9. Serve with wild rice or vegetables of choice.

CHESAPEAKE SHRIMP SALAD

Serves 6

Ingredients

1 tsp peppercorn (whole)*
1 whole bay leaf*
1 lb frozen small shrimp (peeled, shelled, and deveined)
1 clove garlic (minced)
1 tbsp ghee
2 tsp seafood seasoning (divided in two)
2 tbsp mayonnaise (use a light or avocado oil variety)
1 cup celery (chopped)
1 tbsp chopped fresh dill
1 tbsp lemon juice (fresh)
*Use of a spice bag is highly recommended but not required.

Directions

1. Fill a medium-sized pot with water, and bring to a boil.
2. Put whole peppercorns and bay leaf in a spice bag, and add to the boiling water.
3. Next, add shrimp, garlic, ghee, and 1 tsp of seafood seasoning.
4. Boil 1–3 minutes (uncovered) until the shrimp slightly curl up or become opaque.
5. Remove the shrimp from the water using a slotted spoon, or pour shrimp into a strainer. (If you use a spice bag, you won't have to pick out the peppercorns and bay leaf).
6. To a large bowl, add shrimp, mayonnaise, the remaining teaspoon of seafood seasoning, celery, and fresh dill.
7. Add the lemon juice at the end.
8. Mix well.
9. Refrigerate for 30 minutes before enjoying.

CILANTRO CAULIFLOWER RICE

Serves 4

Ingredients

1 large cauliflower
2 tsp olive oil
1/4 cup onion (chopped)
1 clove garlic (minced)
1/2 tsp sea salt
1/4 tsp fresh cracked black pepper
1/2 cup fresh cilantro (divided and stems removed)
2 tbsp ghee
Juice of 1/2 lime

Directions

1. Preheat oven to 425°F.
2. Cut cauliflower into small pieces (hard stems removed), and place in a food processor.
3. Pulse until the cauliflower resembles rice.
4. Place "riced" cauliflower in one even layer on a baking sheet, and bake for 5 minutes. Flip, and bake for 5 minutes more.
5. Remove from oven.
6. In a preheated skillet, add the olive oil.
7. Once the oil is hot, add baked cauliflower rice.
8. Sauté with onion, garlic, salt, pepper, and half the cilantro for 5–10 minutes.
9. Add ghee and fresh lime juice at the last minute of cooking.
10. Mix in the other half of the cilantro.
11. Garnish with lime wedges as desired.

COCONUT CHIA PUDDING

Serves 4

Ingredients

1/2 cup chia seeds
1-1/2 cups coconut milk (unsweetened)
1–2 tbsp maple syrup
1 tbsp vanilla extract
Fresh fruit or nuts for garnish

Directions

1. Pour chia seeds, coconut milk, maple syrup, and vanilla into a large bowl.
2. Mix well.
3. Refrigerate for 2 hours or overnight.
4. Portion as desired.
5. Top with fresh fruits such or nuts.

COCONUT CURRY SHRIMP

Serves 4

Ingredients

1 lb raw shrimp (peeled and deveined)
2 tbsp fresh lime juice
2 tbsp curry powder
1/2 tsp turmeric powder
1 tbsp fresh thyme (stems removed)
1/2 tsp sea salt
1/4 tsp fresh cracked black pepper
1/4 cup red pepper (chopped)
1/4 cup green pepper (chopped)
1/4 tsp all-purpose seasoning
2 cloves garlic (minced)
1 tsp fresh ginger (chopped)
1 Scotch bonnet pepper or habanero (seeds removed unless you like it spicy)
2 tbsp ghee
1–2 tbsp olive oil
13.5 oz coconut milk (unsweetened)

Directions

1. Place raw shrimp in a large bowl.
2. To the bowl add lime juice, curry powder, turmeric, salt, black pepper, red and green peppers, and all-purpose seasoning. Set aside.
3. In a large, preheated skillet (medium heat), sauté garlic, ginger, thyme, and Scotch bonnet pepper in ghee and olive oil.
4. Add coconut milk, and stir together. Let it come to a low boil.
5. Add shrimp to the pot.
6. The shrimp will cook quickly (a few minutes) and will curl once cooked.
7. Remove from heat promptly.
8. Serve hot with sides of your choice (cilantro cauliflower rice is highly recommended).
9. Garnish with additional lime if desired. You may add additional salt and pepper to taste.

COCONUT-LIME CHICKEN

Serves 4

Ingredients

3–5 lbs chicken thighs (cleaned, rinsed, and patted dry)
1/2 tbsp salt (or more to taste)
Fresh cracked black pepper
1 tsp paprika
1/2 tsp granulated garlic
5 sprigs fresh thyme (plus additional for topping)
1 tsp all-purpose seasoning
2 limes (including zest and juice of one lime; slice the other lime thinly)
2 tbsp olive or avocado oil
1/2 cup chicken broth
4 cloves garlic (minced)
1 cup coconut milk (unsweetened)

Directions

1. Season chicken with salt, pepper, paprika, granulated garlic, and all-purpose seasoning.
2. Add lime juice and lime zest, and combine.
3. Let marinate for 2 hours or overnight.
4. Preheat oven to 350°F.
5. To a sauté pan, add oil, and preheat to medium heat.
6. Place chicken skin side down, and brown on each side (about 3–5 minutes per side).
7. Once the chicken is brown, remove and set aside.
8. Drain the oil from the pan, and discard.
9. Return the pan to the heat, and add chicken broth, garlic, thyme, and coconut milk.
10. Cook on low heat for 15 minutes in order to reduce the liquid.
11. Additional salt may be added to taste.
12. Return browned chicken thighs to the pan.
13. Top with sliced lime and additional thyme.
14. Cover the pan, and bake in the oven for 30 minutes.
15. Serve hot with pan gravy.

CREAMY ALMOND PORRIDGE

Serves 8

Ingredients

4 cups blanched or superfine almond flour
1 cup ground flaxseed
1 tbsp ground cinnamon
2 tsp ground nutmeg
5–6 cups unsweetened almond milk
1/2 cup maple syrup
1 tsp vanilla extract

Directions

1. Mix almond flour, flaxseed, cinnamon, and nutmeg in a large bowl.
2. Slowly and steadily add almond milk, and stir gently with a whisk to eliminate any lumps.
3. The amount of milk you add will depend on the thickness you desire.
4. Pour the contents of the bowl into a mid-sized pot on low to medium heat.
5. Be mindful of the temperature so you don't scorch the contents or cause it to bubble and overflow.
6. Add maple syrup and vanilla extract.
7. Continue to stir for a few minutes until heated all the way through.
8. Pour into bowls, and garnish with fruit, nuts, and seeds as desired.

* Note: Use additional milk to reheat any leftovers.

CRISPY SWEET POTATO ROUNDS

Serves 4–6

Ingredients

1 cup olive oil (plus more for drizzling)
2 sweet potatoes, rinsed and cut into 1/4 inch rounds
1 cup cilantro (chopped)
1 tsp salt (1/2 tsp per side)
Fresh cracked black pepper

Directions

1. Preheat oven to 400°F.
2. Drizzle a large sheet pan with some of the olive oil, and evenly distribute it so the pan is lightly oiled.
3. Place sliced sweet potatoes on the oiled sheet pan.
4. In a food processor, blend the rest of the olive oil and the cilantro to make a paste.
5. Using a silicone brush, smear half of the cilantro paste on the first side of the sweet potato rounds.
6. Season the rounds with 1/2 tsp salt and some fresh cracked black pepper.
7. Bake for 20 minutes.
8. Turn over the sweet potato pieces, and spread on the remaining cilantro paste.
9. Sprinkle with the remaining salt and pepper.
10. Bake for 20 minutes more or until golden brown.

CRUNCHY GRAIN-FREE GRANOLA

Serves 6–8

Ingredients

1-1/2 cups almond flour
1-1/2 cups flaked unsweetened coconut
3/4 cup sunflower seeds
3/4 cup pumpkin seeds
3 tbsp vanilla extract
2 tsp ground cinnamon
2 tsp ground nutmeg
1/2 cup maple syrup
1/2–3/4 cup melted coconut oil

Directions

1. Preheat oven to 325°F.
2. Mix all ingredients together, making sure to add the melted coconut oil last.
3. Spread onto a baking sheet.
4. Bake for 15 minutes.
5. Flip mixture over, and bake for 5 minutes more.
6. Let cool before enjoying.
7. Serve with unsweetened almond milk, or use it as a topping for your favorite dairy-free yogurt.

CUCUMBER SALAD

Serves 4

Ingredients

1 cucumber (thinly sliced)
Juice of 1 small lime
3 tbsp extra virgin olive oil
1/2 tsp salt
1/2 tsp minced garlic
1/4 cup red onions (thinly sliced)
1 tsp chopped chives

Directions

1. In a medium-sized bowl, add cucumbers, lime juice, and olive oil.
2. Mix well to coat the cucumbers.
3. Add salt, garlic, red onions, and chives.
4. Stir gently.
5. Refrigerate for at least 15 minutes—the longer, the better. If you can refrigerate overnight in a covered container, that's ideal.
6. Enjoy!

CURRY CHICKEN SALAD

Serves 4–6

Ingredients

(Chicken)

> 3 cups chicken broth or water (enough liquid to cover chicken)
> 3 bay leaves
> 1 tsp whole peppercorns
> 1 tsp salt
> 2 tsp dried tarragon (divided into 2 equal parts)
> 1 tsp fresh thyme
> 3 cloves garlic (chopped)
> 4 boneless chicken thighs (about 2 lbs – cleaned, patted dry, skin and fat removed, cut into 1-inch cubes)
> More salt and pepper to taste
> A spice bag is highly recommended for this recipe

(Dressing)

> 1/2 cup mayonnaise
> 2 tsp curry powder
> 1/3 cup celery (diced)
> 2 tbsp scallions (chopped)
> Freshly cracked black pepper
> Salt to taste
> 1/2 cup green grapes (cut in half)
> 1/2 cup chopped raw walnuts (optional)

Directions

(Chicken)

1. Put chicken broth or water in a pot.
2. If you're using a spice bag, place bay leaves and peppercorns inside, and put in the pot. Otherwise just add them to the pot and remove later.
3. Add salt, half the tarragon, thyme, and garlic.
4. Bring to a boil on medium heat.

5. Poach chicken for about 5 minutes or until cooked all the way through.
6. Let the chicken cool in the refrigerator about 15 minutes.

(Dressing)

1. In a separate bowl, add mayonnaise, curry, celery, scallions, remaining tarragon, and freshly cracked black pepper.
2. Stir to combine with the cooled chicken and more salt to taste.
3. Add grapes and walnuts, and then combine.
4. Let the mixture sit in the refrigerator for at least 2 hours to allow flavors to peak, and enjoy.

EASY EGG SALAD

Serves 4–6

Ingredients

6 hard boiled eggs
2-1/2 tbsp avocado oil mayonnaise
2 tbsp red onion (chopped)
1 tbsp green onion (chopped)
1/2 tsp paprika
1/2 tsp cayenne pepper
Salt and pepper to taste

Directions

1. Peel hard boiled eggs, and mash eggs with a fork.
2. Add mayonnaise, onions, paprika, cayenne, salt, and pepper.
3. Mix well.
4. Let chill in the refrigerator.
5. Serve over greens or watercress.

FLAXSEED QUINOA PORRIDGE

Serves 4

Ingredients

1 cup quinoa
2-1/4 cup almond milk (unsweetened)
2 tbsp maple syrup
1/4 cup ground flaxseed
1 tsp vanilla extract
1 tsp ground cinnamon
Pinch of salt
Blueberries, chopped walnuts, more maple syrup

Directions

1. Cook quinoa according to package instructions. Do not add any additional seasonings or oil.
2. Once the quinoa is cooked, lower the heat, and add almond milk, maple syrup, ground flaxseed, vanilla, cinnamon, and salt to the same pot.
3. Stir intermittently.
4. Cook for 10 minutes until mixture thickens and desired consistency is achieved.
5. Serve with chopped walnuts, blueberries, and a drizzle of maple syrup.

GRAIN-FREE CARROT MUFFINS

Yield: 9

Ingredients

2 cups carrots (shredded)
1/2 cup coconut flakes (unsweetened)
1 cup fine almond flour
1/2 cup tapioca flour
1/2 tsp baking soda
1 tsp ground cinnamon
1/4 tsp ground nutmeg
1/8 tsp sea salt
1 egg (well beaten)
1 tsp vanilla extract
1/4 cup melted coconut oil
1/4 cup almond milk (unsweetened)
1/2 tsp apple cider vinegar
1/4 cup maple syrup
1/4 cup chopped walnuts
1/4 cup raisins
Zest of 1 lemon

Directions

1. Preheat oven to 350°F.
2. In a large bowl, mix carrots, coconut flakes, almond flour, tapioca flour, baking soda, cinnamon, nutmeg, and salt.
3. In another bowl, combine wet ingredients (egg, vanilla, coconut oil, almond milk, apple cider vinegar, maple syrup), and mix well.
4. Slowly add the wet ingredients to the dry ingredients, and stir until combined.
5. Fold in walnuts, raisins, and lemon zest.
6. Line muffin tin with appropriate number of paper liners. (You can also opt to pour the mixture directly into lightly greased muffin tins).
7. Using a ladle or large spoon, fill the tins 3/4 full.
8. Bake 20 minutes.
9. Turn the oven off, and let them sit for 5 minutes.

10. Once baked, a toothpick inserted in the middle should come out clean.
11. Allow muffins to cool completely on a wire rack before enjoying.

GREEN LEAN SCRAMBLE

Serves 4

Ingredients

2 tbsp ghee
1 cup green peppers (chopped)
1 cup broccoli (chopped)
1 cup spinach (fresh or frozen)
1/4 cup green onions (chopped)
10 eggs (well beaten)
3 sprigs fresh thyme (stems removed)
1/2–1 tsp salt (to taste)
1/4 tsp fresh cracked black pepper
Ripe avocados (sliced) (optional)

Directions

1. Preheat a large skillet on medium-low heat.
2. Add 1 tablespoon ghee.
3. Sauté peppers, broccoli, spinach, and green onions.
4. To already beaten eggs, add 1 tbsp water, and whisk.
5. Add the egg mixture to the sautéed vegetables.
6. Add thyme.
7. Cook slowly, up to 10 minutes, constantly stirring to make a scramble.
8. Add the other tablespoon of ghee.
9. Season with salt and black pepper to taste for the last few minutes of cooking.
10. Serve with sliced ripe avocados, if desired.

GREEN ONION HERB SAUCE

Makes 1 cup

Ingredients

4 cloves garlic
3 medium green onions
1/2 Scotch bonnet pepper (seeds removed)
3/4 cup cilantro leaves with stems
1/2 cup parsley leaves
6 tbsp olive oil
1/2 cup red wine vinegar
1/2 tsp salt

Directions

1. Peel and finely mince the garlic.
2. Chop the green onions (both the white and green portions).
3. Mince the Scotch bonnet pepper. For a milder sauce, omit the pepper seeds.
4. Roughly chop the cilantro.
5. Combine the garlic, green onions, Scotch bonnet pepper, cilantro, and parsley in a food processor, and pulse until everything is finely chopped but not blended.
6. Put the mixture in a bowl, and add the olive oil, vinegar, and salt.
7. Whisk to combine.
8. Taste, and add more salt if necessary.
9. Refrigerate before serving.
10. Works well on poultry, beef, lamb, seafood, and eggs.

GREEN PEA SKIN-BRIGHTENING SMOOTHIE

Serves 2

Ingredients

1 banana (frozen)
1 cup green peas (frozen)
1 cup blueberries (frozen)
1 cup coconut milk
1/2 cup coconut water
2 level scoops collagen powder (according to recommended serving)

Directions

1. Put all ingredients in a blender, and mix until smooth.
2. Enjoy!

GRILLED (SOY-FREE) TERIYAKI SALMON

Serves 4

Ingredients

Juice of 1 orange (fresh-squeezed)
1/4 cup coconut aminos
2 garlic cloves (minced)
1 tbsp blackstrap molasses
1 tbsp fresh cilantro (chopped)
1 tbsp ginger (minced)
1/4 tsp red pepper flakes
1 tsp salt
4 pieces wild salmon filets (rinsed and patted dry)
2 tbsp ghee or olive oil
Garnish: sesame seeds, chopped green onions

Directions

1. Mix together fresh-squeezed orange juice, coconut aminos, garlic, molasses, cilantro, ginger, red pepper flakes, and salt.
2. Put salmon filets in a shallow dish.
3. Pour the marinade over the top, and cover.
4. Shake the covered dish, if possible, to allow all the marinade to distribute over the fish.
5. Let marinate for 30 minutes at room temperature.
6. Once marinated, put a skillet on medium heat, and add ghee or olive oil.
7. Once the ghee is melted, add the salmon filets skin side down.
8. Cooking times will vary, but it should take 2 to 4 minutes to cook per side.
9. Flip the salmon, and cook a few minutes more.
10. Do not overcook the salmon.
11. Carefully remove the salmon from the pan, and top with sesame seeds and chopped green onions.
12. If you'd like to serve the salmon with additional teriyaki sauce, heat the sauce on the stove for 3–4 minutes before serving.
13. If not, discard the marinade, and enjoy.

HONEY GINGER BEER

Serves 12

Ingredients

2 hands or 4 medium pieces ginger root
6–10 cups of water (and more to soak)
1 cinnamon stick
4 whole cloves
3/4 cup raw honey
1/2 tsp vanilla extract
Juice of 1 lime

Directions

1. Soak ginger root in enough water to cover for about 30 minutes to loosen the dirt and debris.
2. Discard the water.
3. Lightly scrape the ginger with a knife to remove most of outer skin, and cut into chunks.
4. Add the ginger to a blender with 2 cups water, and pulse to a consistency of grated ginger. It should take only a few seconds.
5. Boil 4 cups water, and pour over the grated ginger.
6. Add the cinnamon stick and whole cloves. Allow the mixture to sit for 2–4 hours until desired potency is achieved. The longer it sits, the stronger the ginger flavor.
7. Use a strainer or sieve to extract the ginger juice from the pulp.
8. Add 2–4 more cups of cold water (depending on your desired taste).
9. Add honey, vanilla, and lime juice, and stir.
10. Serve over ice.
11. Refrigerate any unused ginger beer.

HONEY GINGER SHRIMP

Serves 4

Ingredients

1 lb wild shrimp (peeled and deveined)
Juice of 1 lime
1/4 cup coconut aminos
4 tbsp raw local or Manuka honey
3 cloves garlic (minced)
1/2 tsp salt
1/8 tsp fresh cracked black pepper
1 tbsp ghee or olive oil
Garnish: sesame seeds and sliced scallions

Directions

1. Rinse shrimp with cold water, and pat dry.
2. Place the shrimp in a shallow bowl.
3. In another bowl, add lime juice, coconut aminos, honey, garlic, salt, and pepper.
4. Mix to combine.
5. Pour this marinade over the shrimp, making sure the liquid covers the shrimp.
6. Let the shrimp marinate for 20 minutes, turning half-way through.
7. Preheat a skillet prepared with ghee that has melted.
8. Cook the shrimp for a few minutes per side, making sure not to overcook them.
9. To have additional sauce for serving, heat the reserved marinade in a small saucepan for 2–3 minutes before using.
10. Garnish with scattered sesame seeds and sliced scallions.

ISLAND-STYLE CURRY CHICKEN

Serves 4–6

Ingredients

3 lbs chicken wings (cleaned, rinsed, patted dry, and segmented)
1 tsp allspice (ground)
1 tsp salt
1/2 tsp fresh ground black pepper
1 tsp poultry seasoning
2 tbsp curry powder (divided)
3 garlic cloves (minced)
3 tbsp ghee
1 small onion (diced)
3/4 cup celery (chopped)
4 medium-sized carrots (cut into discs)
1/2 cup red peppers (chopped)
1 tbsp fresh ginger (minced)
5 small potatoes (cubed)
2-1/2 cups chicken broth
1 can coconut milk (13.5 oz)
1 bay leaf
2 whole cloves
6 sprigs fresh thyme
1/2 tsp Scotch bonnet pepper (minced)

Directions

1. Season chicken with allspice, salt, black pepper, poultry seasoning, 1 tbsp curry powder, and minced garlic.
2. Let sit for 1 hour.
3. In a large heavy pot, add 2 tbsp ghee, and preheat on medium heat.
4. Once preheated, brown the chicken a few minutes per side.
5. Remove the chicken, and set aside.
6. Add 1 tbsp ghee.
7. Sauté onions, celery, carrots, peppers, and ginger for 2–3 minutes.
8. Add potatoes, and cook for just 1 minute more.

9. Return the chicken to the pot, and stir in chicken broth, coconut milk, additional 1 tbsp of curry powder, bay leaf, cloves, thyme, and Scotch bonnet pepper.
10. Simmer with lid slightly ajar on medium-low heat for about 45 minutes or until chicken is tender and the gravy has thickened.

KALE MASHED POTATOES

Serves 4–6

Ingredients

6 large russet potatoes (peeled and cut into 1-inch cubes)
Water
3 tsp salt
3 cups kale (rinsed and chopped)
1 clove whole garlic (peeled)
1/2 cup unsweetened macadamia nut milk (can also use other preferred nut milk) – kept warm
Pinch of nutmeg
1/8 tsp fresh cracked black pepper
1 tbsp ghee or olive oil

Directions

1. Place cubed potatoes in a large pot with just enough water to cover.
2. Add 1 tsp salt.
3. Allow it to come to a boil on medium-high heat.
4. Cook until potatoes are fork-tender.
5. Remove the potatoes using a slotted spoon, reserving the water in the pot.
6. To the reserved water, add chopped kale and whole garlic.
7. Cook for 5 minutes, and then remove from heat.
8. Add kale and garlic to a high-speed blender.
9. Add just enough warm macadamia nut milk to blend smoothly.
10. Use a potato masher or ricer to mash the potatoes.
11. Once mashed, add blended kale, milk mixture, and remaining salt.
12. Slowly stir in remaining warm milk a little at a time until you've reached your desired consistency.
13. Add a pinch of nutmeg, cracked pepper, and ghee to finish.

KALE AND MUSHROOM FRITTATA

10 slices

Ingredients

Olive oil
1-1/2 tbsp ghee
1/2 cup red onions (chopped)
2 cloves garlic (minced)
2-1/2 cups kale (rinsed, torn, ribs removed)
1/2 cup mushrooms (chopped) (use a combination of shiitake, porcini, and oyster mushrooms if you can find them; otherwise, use what you have on hand)
1/2 tsp salt (divided)
1 dozen eggs
1/4 cup unsweetened almond or macadamia milk
1 tbsp fresh oregano (torn into pieces)
1/8 tsp cracked black pepper
1 Roma tomato (chopped)
1 tsp dry Italian seasoning
1/4 tsp nutritional yeast flakes
Garnish: herbed olive oil for drizzle and fine sea salt

Directions

1. Preheat oven to 350°F.
2. Place oil in a preheated large (10-inch) skillet on medium-low heat.
3. Melt ghee.
4. Add onions and garlic to the skillet, and simmer for 5 minutes (making sure not to burn them).
5. Tear kale into bite-sized pieces.
6. Sauté kale and mushrooms until tender (about 5 minutes).
7. Season with half the salt.
8. To a large bowl add eggs, almond milk, oregano, pepper, and remaining salt.
9. Beat the mixture until fluffy.
10. Add egg mixture to the preheated skillet.
11. Gently scatter chopped tomato on top.

12. Once eggs begin to firm up around the side of the pan a little, add Italian seasoning and nutritional yeast flakes.
13. Remove from stovetop, and bake about 25 minutes in the preheated oven or until eggs are firm in the middle.
14. Drizzle with herbed olive oil, and sprinkle with fine sea salt as a final touch.

LEMON HERB CHICKEN

Serves 4

Ingredients

2–3 lbs chicken thighs (5–6 pieces cleaned, rinsed, and patted dry)
1/2 tsp salt
1/8 tsp ground black pepper
1 tsp all-purpose seasoning
1 tsp paprika
2 tbsp olive or avocado oil
1 cup chicken broth
1 whole lemon (1/2 sliced, 1/2 juiced)
4 cloves garlic (chopped)
1 tbsp ghee
2 fistfuls fresh thyme (divided in half)

Directions

1. Season chicken with salt, pepper, all-purpose seasoning, and paprika.
2. Let sit for 1 hour.
3. Preheat oven to 350°F.
4. In a large skillet, add oil.
5. Once the skillet is preheated and the oil is hot, brown chicken (about 10 minutes per side).
6. Remove chicken, and set aside.
7. Lower the heat, and add chicken broth and lemon juice to the skillet.
8. Use a wooden spoon to scrape up any bits from the bottom.
9. Add chopped garlic, ghee, and half the thyme.
10. Return chicken to skillet.
11. Top with lemon slices and the other half of the fresh thyme.
12. Cover the skillet, and place it in the preheated oven.
13. Cook for an additional 25 minutes or until juices run clear.
14. Reserve any pan juices for serving.

MANGO BLUEBERRY SALAD

Serves 4

Ingredients

4 cups mixed greens
1 ripe mango (pit removed)
2 cups fresh blueberries
3 tbsp Manuka honey
1/4 cup apple cider vinegar
1/2 cup olive oil or chia oil
Dash of salt
Black pepper to taste
1 cup raw pecans (roughly chopped)

Directions

1. Wash and dry the mixed greens.
2. Cut the mango into chunks, making sure to remove the pit.
3. Wash and dry the blueberries.
4. Place the mango and blueberries in a large bowl with the greens and raw pecans.
5. In a food processor, add honey, apple cider vinegar, oil, salt, pepper and blend.
6. Pour the dressing over the salad.
7. Feel free to add any cooked protein of your choice.
8. Enjoy immediately.

MASHED GREEN BANANAS

Serves 6

Ingredients

6 green bananas
Water
1 cup coconut milk (unsweetened)
2 tbsp ghee
1/2 tsp salt (and more to taste)
1/4 tsp black pepper

Directions

1. Cut off the stems of the bananas.
2. Using a knife, cut the bananas into thirds, leaving the peels on.
3. Place bananas in large pot with enough cold water to cover.
4. Boil on high for 20 minutes or until the green bananas get fork tender.
5. Drain.
6. Allow the bananas to cool slightly before removing the skins.
7. Use a food processor or a fork to mash the bananas into small pieces.
8. In a small pot, warm the coconut milk, ghee, salt, and pepper.
9. Pour the warmed coconut milk mixture into the mashed bananas, and stir.
10. Add more salt and pepper if desired.

MEXICAN-STYLE GRILLED CHICKEN SKEWERS

Serves 4

Ingredients

1 lime (juice and zest)
Juice of 1 orange
2 tbsp olive oil
3–4 garlic cloves (crushed)
2 tbsp blackstrap molasses
1/2 tsp chili powder
1/2 teaspoon ground cumin
1 tsp chipotle peppers (canned)
2–3 sprigs of each parsley and cilantro
1 tsp salt
1/8 tsp fresh cracked black pepper
1 lb skinless boneless chicken breast (cleaned and cut into cubes)
3–6 bell peppers (3 different colors, cut into squares)
1 large onion (cut into squares)
Special tools needed: wooden skewers

Directions

1. Mix lime juice, lime zest, orange juice, oil, garlic, molasses, chili, cumin, chipotle peppers, parsley, cilantro, salt, and pepper.
2. Place the chicken pieces in the marinade (in a resealable bag), and refrigerate for 2–6 hours. I recommend at least 2 hours for optimal flavor.
3. Thread marinated chicken onto wooden skewers, alternating with bell peppers of different colors and onions.
4. Grill on stovetop grill (rotating on alternate sides) until thoroughly cooked.

PERFECT SOFT OR HARD BOILED EGGS

Ingredients

Desired number of eggs (make one layer in the pot; do not pile them up)
Water, enough to just cover the eggs.
Ice (for an ice bath)

Directions

1. Put water in a small to medium-sized pot, and put the heat on high to get the water to a rolling boil.
2. Once the water is boiling, gently add the desired number of eggs to form one layer.
3. Immediately set a timer based on the desired amount of doneness of your boiled eggs.
4. Boil 5–7 minutes for soft boiled.
5. Boil 10–12 minutes for hard boiled.
6. Once the time is up, quickly remove the eggs, and place them in an ice bath for up to 5 minutes.
7. When cracked open, there should be no gray ring around the yolk of the egg.
8. Congratulations! You've cooked a perfectly cooked soft-boiled or hard-boiled egg.

PESTO CHICKEN

Serves 6–8

Ingredients

(Chicken)

2 cups fresh basil
1/2 cup walnuts
Juice of 1/2 lemon
4 cloves garlic (lightly chopped)
1 tsp sea salt
Fresh cracked black pepper to taste
1/2 cup olive oil (plus more for drizzling)
4–6 chicken breasts (cleaned, boneless, and skinless)
2 tbsp ghee

(Garnish)

1/2 lemon (sliced)
4 Roma tomatoes (chopped)
Fresh basil

Directions

(Chicken)

1. Preheat oven to 350°F.
2. Place torn basil, walnuts, lemon juice, garlic, salt, pepper, and olive oil in a food processor.
3. Blend until smooth.
4. Smear mixture over both sides of chicken breasts, and let marinate for 2 hours in a resealable bag.
5. Preheat a cast iron grill to medium heat.
6. Prepare the pan with melted ghee.
7. Grill the chicken 3–5 minutes per side.
8. Try not to move the chicken until you are sure that the grill lines are set, and then flip over.
9. Brush the grill pan with additional ghee between batches of chicken to avoid sticking.
10. Remove the chicken.

11. Place chicken on a flat aluminum sheet pan, and bake in the oven for about 10 minutes or until a meat thermometer placed in the center registers 165°F.
12. Top chicken with the garnish.

(Garnish)

1. Grill the slices of the half lemon in the same cast iron grill as the chicken was cooked in. This step takes 3–5 minutes.
2. Garnish chicken with the grilled lemon slices, fresh chopped Roma tomatoes, and fresh basil.

PINA COLADA SMOOTHIE BOWL

Serves 2–4

Ingredients

2 bananas (frozen)
2 cups pineapple (frozen)
1/2 cup unsweetened almond milk (chilled)
2 tbsp chia seeds
1 cup canned coconut milk (chilled)
3 fresh strawberries (sliced)
1/4 fresh pineapple (sliced)
2 tbsp coconut flakes (unsweetened)

Directions

1. Mix the frozen fruit (bananas, pineapple), almond milk, chia seeds, and coconut milk in a high-speed blender.
2. Blend for 30–45 seconds.
3. Pour into individual bowls, and top with fresh sliced strawberries and pineapple.
4. Sprinkle with unsweetened coconut flakes.

ROASTED CARROTS AND GREEN BEANS

Serves 6

Ingredients

2 tbsp raw honey
1/2 cup water
1/2 tsp red pepper flakes
1 tsp salt (divided in two portions)
1/2 tsp fresh cracked black pepper
1 tsp ginger (minced)
2 tbsp red wine vinegar
6–8 sprigs fresh thyme (stems removed)
3 tbsp olive oil
1 lb carrots (cut across and then lengthwise)
1 lb green beans (trimmed)
2 tsp fresh parsley (chopped)

Directions

1. Preheat oven to 400°F.
2. Place honey, water, pepper flakes, half the salt, ginger, vinegar, and thyme in a pot.
3. Bring to a simmer, and whisk for 10 minutes.
4. Remove from heat.
5. Slowly add olive oil, and mix.
6. On a large sheet pan, place carrots and green beans.
7. Toss the vegetables in the honey-ginger mixture until well coated.
8. Sprinkle with remaining salt and pepper.
9. Bake at 400°F for 20–25 minutes, turning halfway through.
10. Sprinkle with chopped fresh parsley right before serving.

SAUTÉED LEMON KALE

Serves 4

Ingredients

3 cloves garlic (minced)
1/2 cup thinly sliced onions
2 tbsp olive oil
1 bunch chopped kale (rinsed well, center ribs removed)
Juice of 1/2 lemon
1/2 tsp salt
1/4 cup water
1/4 tsp red pepper flakes

Directions

1. In a preheated pan on medium heat, sauté garlic and onions (about 30 seconds) in olive oil and ghee, and then add the kale.
2. Add lemon juice, salt, and water.
3. Cook covered, tossing intermittently until kale is tender, about 10 minutes.
4. Finish by sprinkling with red pepper flakes.

SISSEROU CHICKEN QUINOA SALAD

Serves 8–10

Ingredients

(Salad)

1 lb diced chicken breast
1/4 tsp all-purpose seasoning
1/2 tsp sea salt (portioned in half)
2 tbsp olive oil
1 large red onion (thinly sliced)
1/2 red pepper (cut in short strips)
1 yellow pepper (cut in short strips)
2 cups quinoa (cooked according to package instructions)
1/2 seedless cucumber (chopped)
1 pint grape tomatoes (cut in half)
2 cups green pitted olives
1 ripe mango (diced)
3 tbsp fresh basil (in strips)
1 tbsp dry tarragon
Grilled lemon
Fresh basil

(Dressing)

1 cup extra virgin olive oil
3 tbsp red wine vinegar
1/2 tsp sea salt
2 cloves garlic (minced)
2 tbsp dry Italian seasoning
1/4 tsp fresh cracked black pepper

Directions

(Chicken)

1. Season diced chicken with all-purpose seasoning and half of the salt.
2. Add 2 tbsp olive oil to a grill or sauté pan to preheat.
3. Brown chicken on all sides on medium heat until cooked through.

4. Remove the chicken from the pan.
5. Next, grill red onions and peppers on both sides, adding more oil if needed. Cook for about 10 minutes, and set aside.
6. To a large bowl, add cooked quinoa, cucumber, peppers, onions, grape tomatoes, olives, mango, cooked chicken, basil, and tarragon.

(Dressing)

1. In a food processor, combine olive oil, red wine vinegar, salt, minced garlic, Italian seasoning, and black pepper.
2. Slowly add olive oil while pulsing the food processor.
3. Toss to evenly distribute.
4. Chill dressing for 2 hours (hint: things get merrier the longer they sit), and then add to salad and toss. You can also use the dressing immediately.
5. Garnish with grilled lemon and fresh basil as desired.

SLIM TING VIRGIN ISLANDS POTATO STUFFING

Serves 16

Ingredients

6–8 small to medium sweet potatoes (baked)
1 clove garlic (chopped)
1/2 large yellow onion (chopped)
1/2 red pepper (chopped)
1/4 green pepper (chopped)
1/2 Scotch bonnet or habanero pepper (seeds removed)
3 tbsp fresh thyme (stems removed)
1 cup almond milk (unsweetened)
1 tsp salt
1 cup raisins
1/2 tsp all-purpose seasoning
1 tsp ground cinnamon
1/4 tsp ground nutmeg
1/2 tsp fresh cracked black pepper
2 tbsp maple syrup
Coconut oil spray (for pan)

Directions

1. Preheat oven to 350°F.
2. Remove skin from baked sweet potatoes, and mash well in a large bowl using a fork or potato masher.
3. To a blender add garlic, onions, red pepper, green pepper, Scotch bonnet pepper, and thyme.
4. If you're having a hard time blending the sofrito (garlic, peppers, and onions), add a bit of the almond milk (take from the 1 cup) to help blend it.
5. Put the pureed vegetables in a small pan on medium heat.
6. To the same pan add almond milk, salt, raisins, all-purpose seasoning, cinnamon, and nutmeg.
7. Warm for a few minutes before removing from the heat.
8. Add the seasoned liquid along with the black pepper and maple syrup to the mashed sweet potatoes.
9. Use coconut oil spray to oil a 9x12 pan.

10. Add sweet potato mixture using a rubber scraper to smooth it over.
11. If desired, use the back of a fork to make "happy trails" of the sweet potato stuffing from one end to the other before placing it in the oven.
12. Bake for 45 minutes on the middle rack until golden brown.
13. Allow to cool for 15 minutes before serving.

SPICY BEEF STEW

Serves 10–12

Ingredients

2 lbs beef stew meat (1-inch cubes)
1 tbsp coarse salt
1/2 tsp fresh cracked black pepper
1 tsp multi-purpose seasoning
2 tbsp ghee
1 large yellow onion (chopped)
3 cloves garlic (minced)
2 bay leaves
4 large carrots (sliced)
5 stalks celery (chopped)
1/2 Scotch bonnet or habanero pepper (seeds removed)
1/2 cup wild mushrooms (sliced)
1 (28 oz) can of peeled, whole tomatoes
6 cups beef broth (low sodium)
1 tbsp fresh oregano (chopped)
1 tsp fresh rosemary (leaves or needles only)
1 tsp fresh thyme (stems removed)
1/2 tsp cloves
5 medium-sized potatoes (cubed)
1 tbsp dried parsley

Directions

1. Season the beef with salt, black pepper, and all-purpose seasoning.
2. Place the ghee in a large Dutch oven on low to medium-low heat.
3. In small batches, brown meat on all sides until it forms a nice crust, adding more ghee if needed.
4. Remove the meat, and put it on a large plate.
5. Add onions, garlic, and bay leaves.
6. Cook on low heat for 5 minutes.
7. To the same pot add carrots, celery, Scotch bonnet or habanero pepper, and mushrooms.
8. Simmer on low for an additional 10 minutes, making sure to stir often.

9. Remove the contents from the pot, and set aside.
10. To the same pot add the beef broth.
11. Use a wooden spoon to scrape up any remaining bits from the bottom of the pan.
12. Break up the whole tomatoes into chunks, and add to the beef broth.
13. Return beef to the pot, and add oregano, rosemary, thyme, and cloves.
14. Simmer slowly on low for 1-1/2 hours.
15. Return the simmered veggies to the pot.
16. Add potatoes, and cook slowly on low for an additional 1-1/2 hours.
17. Remove bay leaves.
18. Top with dried parsley just before serving.

STEW PAPAYA

Serves 4

Ingredients

1/2 green papaya (cut into small pieces)
1 cup coconut milk (unsweetened)
1 tbsp ghee
1/2 tsp ground allspice
1/2 tsp salt
1/2 tsp fresh cracked black pepper

Directions

1. Add papaya, coconut milk, ghee, allspice, and salt and pepper to a small saucepan.
2. Cook covered on medium-low heat for about 20 minutes or until fork-tender.
3. Serve warm.

TRAFALGAR TROPICAL SMOOTHIE

Serves 4

Ingredients

2 cups ripe papaya (seeds removed)
1 ripe banana (frozen)
1 cup diced mango (frozen)
1 can (13.5 oz) chilled coconut milk (unsweetened)
1 tsp vanilla extract

Directions

1. Add all the ingredients to a blender, and combine until smooth.
2. Pour, and enjoy immediately.

WARM DIJON POTATO SALAD WITH CARAMELIZED ONIONS

Serves 6–8

Ingredients

2 lbs small red potatoes (cut into equal bite-sized pieces)
Water
1 tsp salt (plus more to taste)
2 tbsp ghee or unsalted butter
1/2 large sweet onion (sliced thinly)
2 tbsp Dijon mustard
2 tbsp red wine vinegar
2 tbsp fresh oregano
1 clove garlic (chopped)
1/8 tsp fresh cracked black pepper
1/4 cup extra virgin olive oil
Zest of 1 lemon
1 tbsp fresh dill

Directions

1. Put potatoes in a large pot with just enough water to cover them.
2. Add salt, and cook on medium-high heat until fork-tender.
3. Drain well.
4. Add butter to a skillet along with the sliced onions.
5. Cook onion slices on low heat for about 45 minutes, stirring frequently until they are soft and brown (caramelized). Remove from heat.
6. To a food processor add mustard, vinegar, oregano, garlic, pepper, and salt to taste.
7. Stream in olive oil a little at a time, pulsing intermittently.
8. Pour dressing over cooked potatoes, and add caramelized onions.
9. Stir well.
10. Top with lemon zest and chopped dill right before serving.

IN GRATITUDE

Thanks, Mom (Jeanillia), for risking it all and moving to another country, land unseen, on faith and a prayer. Without your sacrifice, I wouldn't be where I am today.

Big love to triple B—Bryan, Brylee, and Bali. I couldn't do this without you. I mean I probably could, but this is the kind of stuff you're supposed to say in the gratitude section. Love you like plantain.

FURTHER READING

Chapter 7: The Grocery Game

Center for Food Safety and Applied Nutrition. "GMO Crops, Animal Food, and Beyond." U.S. Food and Drug Administration, FDA. *https://www.fda. gov/food/agricultural-biotechnology/gmo-crops-animal-food-and-beyond#:~:text=Corn percent20is percent20the percent20most percent20commonly, percent2C percent20livestock percent2C percent20or percent20other percent20animals*

Rueda-Ruzafa, L; Cruz, F; Roman, P; Cardona, D. "Gut Microbiota and Neurological Effects of Glyphosate." Neurotoxicology, U.S. National Library of Medicine.

https://pubmed.ncbi.nlm.nih.gov/31442459/

The Nutrition Source. "Lectins." The Nutrition Source, 2 Mar. 2022. *https:// www.hsph.harvard.edu/nutritionsource/anti-nutrients/lectins*

Thompson, Tricia, et al. "Lentils and Gluten Cross Contact." Frontiers in Nutrition, U.S. National Library of Medicine, 29 Apr. 2022. *https:// www.ncbi.nlm.nih.gov/pmc/articles/PMC9101047/#:~:text=Lentils percent20are percent20naturally percent20gluten percent2Dfree.,contact percent20with percent20gluten percent2Dcontaining percent20grains*

Chapter 8: Food—The Good and Bad

Beyond Celiac. "Celiac Disease: Fast Facts." Beyond Celiac, 14 Nov. 2022. *https://www.beyondceliac.org/celiac-disease/facts-and-figures/#:~:text=An percent20estimated percent201 percent20in percent20133,celiac percent20disease percent20to percent20be percent201.6 percent25*

Center for Food Safety and Applied Nutrition. "How to Understand and Use the Nutrition Facts Label." U.S. Food and Drug Administration. *https://www.fda.gov/food/new-nutrition-facts-label/ how-understand-and-use-nutrition-facts-label*

Klein, Ned. "Exemption from Nutrition Labeling Requirements." FDA Reader, 21 Nov. 2022. *https://www.fdareader.com/blog/2018/12/11/exemption-from-food-labeling-requirements percentEF percentBB percentBF*

Vojdani, Aristo and Tarash, Igal. "Cross-Reaction between Gliadin and Different Food and Tissue Antigens." Food and Nutrition Sciences, Scientific Research Publishing, 10 Jan. 2013. *https://www.scirp.org/journal/PaperInformation.aspx?PaperID=26626*

Chapter 9: Fiber Filled

Board, Mango. "Fiber from Mangos." Mango.org, 9 Apr. 2021. *https://www.mango.org/blog-fiber-from-mangos/#:~:text=A percent203 percent2F4 percent20cup percent20*

DGA.gov. "Current Dietary Guidelines." Food Sources of Dietary Fiber | Dietary Guidelines for Americans. *https://www.dietaryguidelines.gov/resources/2020-2025-dietary-guidelines-online-materials/food-sources-select-nutrients/food-0*

FoodData Central. "Fooddata Central Search Results." FoodData Central. *https://fdc.nal.usda.gov/fdc-app.html#/food-details/170151/nutrients*

McManus, Katherine D. "Should I Be Eating More Fiber?" Harvard Health, 27 Feb. 2019. *https://www.health.harvard.edu/blog/should-i-be-eating-more-fiber-2019022115927*

The Nutrition Source. "Quinoa." The Nutrition Source, 6 July 2021. *https://www.hsph.harvard.edu/nutritionsource/food-features/quinoa/#:~:text=Though percent20technically percent20a percent20seed percent2C percent20Quinoa,and percent205 percent20grams percent20of percent20fiber*

Pereira, MA; O'Reilly, E; Augustasson K; et al. Archives of Internal Medicine. "Dietary and Coronary Fiber Heart Disease: A Pooled Analysis of Cohort Studies." Arc of Internal Med 2004; 164: 370-6.

Sawada, N; Iwasaki, M; Yamaji, T; Shimazu, T; Sasazuki, S; Inoue, M; Tsugane, S. "Fiber Intake and Risk of Subsequent Prostate Cancer in Japanese Men." The American Journal of Clinical Nutrition, U.S. National Library of Medicine. *https://pubmed.ncbi.nlm.nih.gov/25527755*

Whitbread, Daisy. "29 Fruits High in Fiber." Myfooddata, My Food Data, 27 Sept. 2022. *https://www.myfooddata.com/articles/fruits-high-in-fiber.php*

Chapter 10: Be Plantiful!

Buendia, I; Michalska, P; Navarro, E; Gameiro, I; Egea, J; León, R. "Nrf2-Are Pathway: An Emerging Target against Oxidative Stress and Neuroinflammation in Neurodegenerative Diseases." Pharmacology & Therapeutics, U.S. National Library of Medicine. *https://pubmed.ncbi.nlm.nih.gov/26617217/#:~:text=The percent20Nrf2 percent2DARE percent20pathway percent20is,of percent20cytoprotective percent20and percent20detoxificant percent20genes*

Dinkova-Kostova, Albena T, et al. "Keap1 And Done? Targeting the NRF2 Pathway with Sulforaphane." Trends in Food Science & Technology, U.S. National Library of Medicine, Nov. 2017, *https://www.ncbi.nlm.nih.gov/pmc/articles/PMC5725197/*

Chapter 11: Oh, Sugar Sugar!

Mäkinen, Kauko K. "Gastrointestinal Disturbances Associated with the Consumption of Sugar Alcohols with Special Consideration of Xylitol: Scientific Review and Instructions for Dentists and Other Health-Care Professionals." International Journal of Dentistry, U.S. National Library of Medicine, 2016, *https://www.ncbi.nlm.nih.gov/pmc/articles/PMC5093271*

Reedy, Julia, "How the U.S. Low-Fat Diet Recommendations of 1977 Contributed to the Declining Health of Americans" (2016). Honors Scholar Theses. 490.

UCSF. "Hidden in Plain Sight." SugarScience. UCSF.edu, 7 Dec. 2018. *https://sugarscience.ucsf.edu/hidden-in-plain-sight/#.Y7Sjc3bMI2y*

Witkowski, Marco, et al. "The Artificial Sweetener Erythritol and Cardiovascular Event Risk." Nature News, Nature Publishing Group, 27 Feb. 2023. *https://www.nature.com/articles/s41591-023-02223-9.*

Chapter 12: Big Fat Lies

Brown, Mary Jane. "Advanced Glycation End Products (Ages): A Complete Overview." Healthline, Healthline Media, 22 Oct. 2019. *https://www.healthline.com/nutrition/advanced-glycation-end-products*

McNamara, Donald J. "The Fifty Year Rehabilitation of the Egg." Nutrients, U.S. National Library of Medicine, 21 Oct. 2015. *https://www.ncbi.nlm.nih.gov/pmc/articles/PMC4632449*

Oregon State Univ. "Essential Fatty Acids." Linus Pauling Institute, 14 Mar. 2022. *https://lpi.oregonstate.edu/mic/other-nutrients/essential-fatty-acids*

Pereira, MA; O'Reilly, E; Augustasson, K; et al. Archives of Internal Medicine. "Dietary and Coronary Fiber Heart Disease: A Pooled Analysis of Cohort Studies." Arc of Internal Med 2004; 164: 370-6.

Réhault-Godbert, Sophie, et al. "The Golden Egg: Nutritional Value, Bioactivities, and Emerging Benefits for Human Health." Nutrients, U.S. National Library of Medicine, 22 Mar. 2019. *https://www.ncbi.nlm.nih.gov/ pmc/articles/PMC6470839*

Rungratanawanich, Wiramon, et al. "Advanced Glycation End Products (AGES) and Other Adducts in Aging-Related Diseases and Alcohol-Mediated Tissue Injury." Nature News, Nature Publishing Group, 10 Feb. 2021. *https://www.nature.com/articles/s12276-021-00561-7*

Taha, Ameer Y. "Linoleic Acid–Good or Bad for the Brain?" Nature News, Nature Publishing Group, 2 Jan. 2020. *https://www.nature.com/articles/ s41538-019-0061-9*

Zahed, Rahmin. "9 Health Benefits of Eating Eggs for Breakfast." Keck Medicine of USC, 23 Nov. 2022. *https://www.keckmedicine.org/ blog/10-healthy-benefits-of-eating-eggs-for-breakfast/#:~:text=Eating percent-t2Oeggs percent2Oleads percent2Oto percent2Oelevated,increased percent2OHDL percent2Olevels percent2Oby percent2O10 percent25*

Chapter 14: Food Breaks

Editors, Fast Times. "20 Facts about Fasting (Backed by Science)." Fasting.com, 7 Jan. 2021. *https://fasting.com/ fast-facts/20-facts-about-fasting-backed-by-science*

Jay, Summer. "The Benefits of Intermittent Fasting for Sleep." Sleep Foundation, 24 June 2022. *https://www.sleepfoundation.org/physical-health/ intermittent-fasting-sleep*

Manoogian, Emily N C, et al. "Time-restricted Eating for the Prevention and Management of Metabolic Diseases," Endocrine Reviews, Volume 43, Issue 2, April 2022, Pages 405–436. *https://doi.org/10.1210/endrev/bnab027*

NMN.com. "What Is Nad+?: Why Is It Important for Health and Longevity?" NMN.com. *https://www.nmn.com/precursors/what-is-nad*

Sruthi, M. "What Happens to Your Body When You Fast for 16 Hours? 16:8 Diet." MedicineNet, MedicineNet, 21 Dec. 2021. *https://www.medicinenet.com/what_happens_to_you_when_you_fast_for_16_hours/article.htm*

Phillips, Matthew. "Fasting as a Therapy in Neurological Disease." Nutrients, U.S. National Library of Medicine. *https://pubmed.ncbi.nlm.nih.gov/31627405*

Patel, Sumit, et al. "1354-P: Alternate-Day Intermittent Fasting Improves Diabetes and Protects Beta-Cell Function in Polygenic Mouse Models of T2DM." American Diabetes Association, American Diabetes Association, 1 June 2022. *https://diabetesjournals.org/diabetes/article/71/Supplement_1/1354-P/146766/1354-P-Alternate-Day-Intermittent-Fasting-Improves*

Rees, Mathieu. "Autophagy: Definition, Health Effects, Fasting, and More." Medical News Today, MediLexicon International. *https://www.medicalnewstoday.com/articles/autophagy*

Tagde, Priti, et al. "Multifaceted Effects of Intermittent Fasting on the Treatment and Prevention of Diabetes, Cancer, Obesity, or Other Chronic Diseases," Current Diabetes Reviews. *https://www.ingentaconnect.com/content/ben/cdr/2022/00000018/00000009/art00004*

Chapter 16: Inflammaging and Healthspan

Baliga, Manjeshwar and Dsouza, Jason. "Amla (Emblica Officinalis Gaertn), a Wonder Berry in the Treatment and Prevention of Cancer." European Journal of Cancer Prevention: The Official Journal of the European Cancer Prevention Organisation (ECP), U.S. National Library of Medicine. *https://pubmed.ncbi.nlm.nih.gov/21317655/*

GreenMedInfo. "Effect of Cinnamon Supplementation on Blood Pressure and Anthropometric Parameters in Patients with Type 2 Diabetes: A Systematic Review and Meta-Analysis of Clinical Trials." *https://greenmedinfo.com/article/cinnamon-supplementation-significantly-decreased-systolic-blood-pressure-and-d*

Gunawardena, D, et al. "Anti-Inflammatory Activity of Cinnamon (C. Zeylanicum and C. Cassia) Extracts - Identification of e-Cinnamaldehyde and O-Methoxy Cinnamaldehyde as the Most Potent Bioactive Compounds." Food & Function, U.S. National Library of Medicine. *https://pubmed.ncbi.nlm.nih.gov/25629927*

Hayward, Nicholas J, et al. "Cinnamon Shows Antidiabetic Properties That Are Species-Specific: Effects on Enzyme Activity Inhibition and Starch Digestion." Plant Foods for Human Nutrition (Dordrecht, Netherlands), U.S. National Library of Medicine, Dec. 2019. *https://www.ncbi.nlm.nih.gov/pmc/articles/PMC6900266/*

Kaputk. "5 Health Benefits of Cayenne Pepper." Cleveland Clinic, Cleveland Clinic, 8 Dec. 2022. *https://health.clevelandclinic.org/cayenne-pepper-benefits/*

Li, Hailong, et al. "Evaluation of the Chemical Composition, Antioxidant and Anti-Inflammatory Activities of Distillate and Residue Fractions of Sweet Basil Essential Oil," J Food Sci Tecnol. *https://www.ncbi.nlm.nih.gov/pmc/articles/PMC5495712/*

Schafer, Georgia, et al. " The Immunomodulation and Anti-Inflammatory Effects of Garlic Organosulfur Compounds in Cancer Chemoprevention," Anticancer Agents Med Chem. *https://www.ncbi.nlm.nih.gov/pmc/articles/PMC3915757/*

URMC. "Ginger." University of Rochester Medical Center. *https://www.urmc.rochester.edu/encyclopedia/content.aspx?contenttypeid=19&contentid=Ginger*

Chapter 17: You're Such a Teas

Mousavi, Ateke, et al. "The Effects of Green Tea Consumption on Metabolic and Anthropometric Indices in Patients with Type 2 Diabetes." Journal of Research in Medical Sciences: the Official Journal of Isfahan University of Medical Sciences, U.S. National Library of Medicine, Dec. 2013. *https://www.ncbi.nlm.nih.gov/pmc/articles/PMC3908530*

Uspenski, Maria. Cancer Hates Tea: A Unique Preventive and Transformative Lifestyle Change to Help Crush Cancer. Page Street Publishing Co., 2016.

Chapter 18: It's Time for a Gut Check

Looi, Mun-Keat. "The Human Microbiome: Everything You Need to Know about the 39 Trillion Microbes That Call Our Bodies Home." Human Microbiome: 39 Trillion Microbes and Bacteria That Call Us Home | BBC Science Focus Magazine, BBC Science Focus Magazine, 14 July 2020. *https://www.sciencefocus.com/the-human-body/human-microbiome/*

Mercola, Dr. Joseph, et al. "MIT Scientist: How Glyphosate Destroys Your Health." Children's Health Defense, 30 June 2021. *https://childrenshealthdefense. org/defender/stephanie-seneff-toxic-legacy-glyphosate-destroying-our-health/*

Miller, Korin. "6 Sneaky Reasons Collagen Declines + How to Support It Naturally*." Mindbodygreen, Mindbodygreen, 26 Aug. 2021. *https://www.mindbodygreen.com/articles/ the-reasons-collagen-declines-how-to-support-it-naturally*

Mu, Qinghui, et al. "Leaky Gut as a Danger Signal for Autoimmune Diseases." Frontiers in Immunology, U.S. National Library of Medicine, 23 May 2017. *https://www.ncbi.nlm.nih.gov/pmc/articles/PMC5440529*

Rueda-Ruzafa, L; Cruz, F; Roman, P; Cardona, D. "Gut Microbiota and Neurological Effects of Glyphosate." Neurotoxicology, U.S. National Library of Medicine. *https://pubmed.ncbi.nlm.nih.gov/31442459*

Chapter 19: Mineral Mastery

American Osteopathic Association. "Low magnesium levels make vitamin D ineffective: Up to 50 percent of US population is magnesium deficient." ScienceDaily. ScienceDaily, 26 February 2018. *https://www.sciencedaily.com/ releases/2018/02/180226122548.htm*

Barbagallo, Mario, and Dominguez, Ligia J. "Magnesium and Type 2 Diabetes." World Journal of Diabetes, U.S. National Library of Medicine, 25 Aug. 2015. *https://www.ncbi.nlm.nih.gov/pmc/articles/PMC4549665*

Center for Food Safety and Applied Nutrition. "Qualified Health Claim Magnesium Reduced Risk of High Blood Pressure." U.S. Food and Drug Administration. *https://www.fda.gov/food/cfsan-constituent-updates/ fda-announces-qualified-health-claim-magnesium-and-reduced-risk-high-blood-pressure*

Chesak, Jennifer. "Supplementing with This Mineral Can Help Keep Blood Sugar Levels in Check." Mindbodygreen, 17 Sept. 2021. *https://www. mindbodygreen.com/articles/magnesium-for-blood-sugar*

Cleveland Clinic. "Magnesium-Rich Food Information." Cleveland Clinic. *https://my.clevelandclinic.org/health/articles/15650-magnesium-rich-food*

DiNicolantonio, James J, et al. "Subclinical Magnesium Deficiency: A Principal Driver of Cardiovascular Disease and a Public

Health Crisis." Open Heart, Archives of Disease in Childhood, 1 Jan. 2018. *https://openheart.bmj.com/content/5/1/e000668.*

Drutel, Anne, et al. "Selenium and the Thyroid Gland: More Good News for Clinicians." Clinical Endocrinology, U.S. National Library of Medicine. *https://pubmed.ncbi.nlm.nih.gov/23046013*

Food Struct. "Brazil Nut vs Apple - in-Depth Nutrition Comparison." Food Struct. *https://foodstruct.com/compare/nuts-brazilnuts-dried-unblanched-vs-apples*

Fukushima, T; Horike, H; Fujiki, S; Kitada, S; Sasaki, T; Kashihara, N. "Zinc Deficiency Anemia and Effects of Zinc Therapy in Maintenance Hemodialysis Patients." Therapeutic Apheresis and Dialysis : Official Peer-Reviewed Journal of the International Society for Apheresis, the Japanese Society for Apheresis, the Japanese Society for Dialysis Therapy, U.S. National Library of Medicine. *https://pubmed.ncbi.nlm.nih. gov/19527468/#:~:text=Zinc percent20concentration percent20and percent20all percent20anemia,highest percent20value percent20at percent203 percent20weeks*

Healthwise Staff. "Getting Enough Calcium and Vitamin D." Michigan Medicine, 9 May 2022. *https://www.uofmhealth.org/health-library/za1487*

Hill, Ansley. "10 Interesting Types of Magnesium (and What to Use Each for)." Healthline Media, 12 July 2022. *https://www.healthline.com/nutrition/magnesium-types#_noHeaderPrefixedContent*

Institute of Medicine (US) Committee on Use of Dietary Reference Intakes in Nutrition Labeling. "A Brief Review of the History and Concepts of the History and Concepts of the Dietary Reference Intakes." Washington (DC): National Academies Press (US); 2003. *https://www.ncbi. nlm.nih.gov/books/NBK208878/*

Kostov, Krasimir. "Effects of Magnesium Deficiency on Mechanisms of Insulin Resistance in Type 2 Diabetes: Focusing on the Processes of Insulin Secretion and Signaling." Multidisciplinary Digital Publishing Institute, 18 Mar. 2019. *https://www.mdpi.com/1422-0067/20/6/1351*

The Nutrition Source. "Magnesium." The Nutrition Source, 14 Oct. 2021. *https://www.hsph.harvard.edu/nutritionsource/magnesium*

The Nutrition Source. "Zinc." The Nutrition Source, 2 Mar. 2022. *https://www.hsph.harvard.edu/nutritionsource/zinc/#:~:text=Zinc percent20is percent20a percent20trace percent20mineral,supporting percent20a percent-20healthy percent20immune percent20system*

Negro, Roberto. "Selenium and Thyroid Autoimmunity." Biologics : Targets & Therapy, U.S. National Library of Medicine, June 2008. *https://www.ncbi.nlm.nih.gov/pmc/articles/PMC2721352*

News-Medical.Net. "Magnesium Essential for Absorption and Metabolism of Vitamin D and Calcium." News-Medical.Net, 19 June 2019. *https://www.news-medical.net/news/20110615/Magnesium-essential-for-absorption-and-metabolism-of-vitamin-D-and-calcium.aspx#:~:text= percent22Adequate percent20levels percent20of percent20magnesium percent20in,it percent20can percent20help percent20calcium percent20absorption*

NIH Office of Dietary Supplements. "Zinc." NIH Office of Dietary Supplements, U.S. Department of Health and Human Services. *https://ods.od.nih.gov/factsheets/Zinc-Consumer*

Park, Hoon, et al. "The Therapeutic Effect and the Changed Serum Zinc Level after Zinc Supplementation in Alopecia Areata Patients Who Had a Low Serum Zinc Level." Annals of Dermatology, U.S. National Library of Medicine, May 2009. *https://www.ncbi.nlm.nih.gov/pmc/articles/PMC2861201*

Patel, Sumit, et al. "1354-P: Alternate-Day Intermittent Fasting Improves Diabetes and Protects Beta-Cell Function in Polygenic Mouse Models of T2DM." American Diabetes Association, American Diabetes Association, 1 June 2022. *https://diabetesjournals.org/diabetes/article/71/Supplement_1/1354-P/146766/1354-P-Alternate-Day-Intermittent-Fasting-Improves*

Pereira, Meire Ellen, et al. "Effects of Selenium Supplementation in Patients with Mild Cognitive Impairment or Alzheimer's Disease: A Systematic Review and Meta-Analysis." Nutrients, U.S. National Library of Medicine, 5 Aug. 2022. *https://www.ncbi.nlm.nih.gov/pmc/articles/PMC9370215*

Petre, Alina. "Top 10 Vegan Sources of Calcium." Healthline, Healthline Media, 13 Mar. 2019. *https://www.healthline.com/nutrition/vegan-calcium-sources#3.-Certain-Nuts*

Prance, G.T. "Brazil Nuts." Encyclopedia of Food Sciences and Nutrition (Second Edition), Academic Press, 6 Dec 2003, Pages 615-619, ISBN 9780122270550.

https://doi.org/10.1016/B0-12-227055-X/00119-X

https://www.sciencedirect.com/science/article/pii/B012227055X00119X

Razavi, M., et al. "Selenium Supplementation and the Effects on Reproductive Outcomes, Biomarkers of Inflammation, and Oxidative Stress in Women with Polycystic Ovary Syndrome." Hormone and Metabolic Research = Hormon- Und Stoffwechselforschung = Hormones Et Metabolisme, U.S. National Library of Medicine. *https://pubmed.ncbi. nlm.nih.gov/26267328*

Ruggeri, Christine. "Top 17 Foods High in Zinc and Their Health Benefits." Dr. Axe, 23 Mar. 2022. *https://draxe.com/nutrition/foods-high-in-zinc*

Scavo, Simone, and Oliven, Valentina. "Zinc Ionophores: Chemistry and Biological Applications." Journal of Inorganic Biochemistry, U.S. National Library of Medicine. *https://pubmed.ncbi.nlm.nih.gov/34929542*

Scientific American. "Diet Poor: Have Fruits and Vegetables Become Less Nutritious?" Scientific American. *https://www.scientificamerican.com/ article/soil-depletion-and-nutrition-loss/#:~:text=The percent20main percent-20culprit percent20in percent20this,the percent20food percent20we percent20eat percent20grows.*

Sherrell, Zia. "Types of Magnesium: Differences, Benefits, and Side Effects." Medical News Today, MediLexicon International, 22 Mar. 2021. *https://www.medicalnewstoday.com/articles/types-of-magnesium*

Stockler-Pinto, et al. "Effect of Selenium Supplementation via Brazil Nut (Bertholletia Excelsa, HBK) on Thyroid Hormones Levels in Hemodialysis Patients: A Pilot Study." Nutricion Hospitalaria, U.S. National Library of Medicine. *https://pubmed.ncbi.nlm.nih.gov/26545554*

Tarleton, B. "Magnesium Intake and Depression in Adults." Journal of the American Board of Family Medicine: JABFM, U.S. National Library of Medicine. *https://pubmed.ncbi.nlm.nih.gov/25748766*

Whitbread, Daisy. "Top 10 Fruits Highest in Magnesium." My Food Data, 27 Sept. 2022. *https://www.myfooddata.com/articles/high-magnesium-fruits.php*

Workinger, Jayme L, et al. "Challenges in the Diagnosis of Magnesium Status." Nutrients, U.S. National Library of Medicine, 1 Sept. 2018. *https:// www.ncbi.nlm.nih.gov/pmc/articles/PMC6163803*

Chapter 20: Vital Vitamins

Brzezińska, Olga, et al. "Role of Vitamin C in Osteoporosis Development and Treatment-A Literature Review." Nutrients, U.S. National Library of Medicine, 10 Aug. 2020. *https://www.ncbi.nlm.nih.gov/pmc/articles/ PMC7469000*

Dawson-Hughes, Bess, et al. "Estimates of Optimal Vitamin D Status - Osteoporosis International." SpringerLink, Springer-Verlag, 18 Mar. 2005. *https://link.springer.com/article/10.1007/s00198-005-1867-7*

Din, U.S.U, et al. "A Double-Blind Placebo Controlled Trial into the Impacts of HMB Supplementation and Exercise on Free-Living Muscle Protein Synthesis, Muscle Mass and Function, in Older Adults." Clinical Nutrition, Volume 38, Issue 5, Sept 2019, Pages 2071-2078.

https://doi.org/10.1016/j.clnu.2018.09.025.

https://www.sciencedirect.com/science/article/pii/S0261561418324634

Harvard Health. "Age and Muscle Loss." Harvard Health, 11 Nov. 2021. *https://www.health.harvard.edu/exercise-and-fitness/age-and-muscle-loss*

Harvard University. "Vitamin D." The Nutrition Source, 14 Nov. 2022. *https://www.hsph.harvard.edu/nutritionsource/vitamin-d*

Lena, Alessia, et al. "Muscle Wasting and Sarcopenia in Heart Failure-the Current State of Science." International Journal of Molecular Sciences, U.S. National Library of Medicine, 8 Sept. 2020. *https://www.ncbi.nlm.nih. gov/pmc/articles/PMC7555939*

Lynch, SR, and Cook, JD. "Interaction of Vitamin C and Iron." Annals of the New York Academy of Sciences, U.S. National Library of Medicine. *https://pubmed.ncbi.nlm.nih.gov/6940487*

Miljkovic, Iva, et al. "Low Prevalence of Vitamin D Deficiency in Elderly Afro-Caribbean Men." Ethnicity & Disease, U.S. National Library of Medicine, 2011. *https://www.ncbi.nlm.nih.gov/pmc/articles/PMC3095488*

More, Daniel. "A Vitamin D Deficiency Can Make Your Allergies Worse." Verywell Health, Verywell Health, 29 Aug. 2021. *https://www.verywellhealth. com/vitamin-d-deficiency-causes-asthma-and-allergies-83031#citation-2*

Office of Dietary Supplements. "Vitamin D." NIH Office of Dietary Supplements, U.S. Department of Health and Human Services, *https://ods.od.nih.gov/factsheets/vitamind-healthprofessional*

Penckofer, Sue, et al. "Vitamin D and Diabetes: Let the Sunshine In." The Diabetes Educator, U.S. National Library of Medicine, 2008. *https://www.ncbi.nlm.nih.gov/pmc/articles/PMC2910714*

Staud, Roland. "Vitamin D: More than Just Affecting Calcium and Bone." Current Rheumatology Reports, U.S. National Library of Medicine. *https://pubmed.ncbi.nlm.nih.gov/16174483*

Uchitomi, Ran, et al. "Vitamin D and Sarcopenia: Potential of Vitamin D Supplementation in Sarcopenia Prevention and Treatment." Nutrients, U.S. National Library of Medicine, 19 Oct. 2020. *https://www.ncbi.nlm.nih.gov/pmc/articles/PMC7603112*

University of Manchester. "Midday Sun Holds The Key To Good Health." ScienceDaily. ScienceDaily, 26 May 2005. *www.sciencedaily.com/releases/2005/05/050526091912.htm*

Wacker, Matthias, and Holick, Michael F. "Sunlight and Vitamin D: A Global Perspective for Health." Dermato-Endocrinology, U.S. National Library of Medicine, 1 Jan. 2013. *https://www.ncbi.nlm.nih.gov/pmc/articles/PMC3897598*

Wimalawansa, Sunil, et al. "Calcium and Vitamin D in Human Health: Hype or Real?" The Journal of Steroid Biochemistry and Molecular Biology, Pergamon, 16 Dec. 2017. *https://www.sciencedirect.com/science/article/abs/pii/S0960076017303813*

Chapter 21: Inside the Caribbean Market

FoodData Central. "Fooddata Central Search Results." FoodData Central. *https://fdc.nal.usda.gov/fdc-app.html#/food-details/167763/nutrients*

Mango.org."Mango Nutrition." Mango.org, 28 Feb. 2022. *https://www.mango.org/mango-nutrition*

WebMD Editorial Contributors. "Soursop: Health Benefits, Nutrients per Serving, Preparation Information and More." WebMD. *https://www.webmd.com/food-recipes/health-benefits-soursop*

Chapter 22: Natural Medicine Cabinet

Beheshti, Zahra, et al. "Influence of apple cider vinegar on blood lipids." Life Science Journal 9 (2012). *https://www.researchgate.net/publication/260311324_Influence_of_apple_cider_vinegar_on_blood_lipids*

Brands, Michael. "Role of Insulin-Mediated Antinatriuresis in Sodium Homeostasis and Hypertension." AHA Journals. *https://www.ahajournals.org/doi/10.1161/HYPERTENSIONAHA.118.11728*

Cohen, Hillel W, et al. "Sodium Intake and Mortality in the NHANES II Follow-up Study." The American Journal of Medicine, Elsevier, 1 Mar. 2006. *https://www.amjmed.com/article/S0002-9343(05)01046-6/fulltext*

DiNicolantonio, James J, and Lucan, Sean C. "The Wrong White Crystals: Not Salt but Sugar as Aetiological in Hypertension and Cardiometabolic Disease." Open Heart, Archives of Disease in Childhood, 1 Nov. 2014. *https://openheart.bmj.com/content/1/1/e000167*

Hadi, Amir, et al. "The Effect of Apple Cider Vinegar on Lipid Profiles and Glycemic Parameters: A Systematic Review and Meta-Analysis of Randomized Clinical Trials - BMC Complementary Medicine and Therapies." SpringerLink, BioMed Central, 29 June 2021, *https://link.springer.com/article/10.1186/s12906-021-03351-w*

Jain, Rahi et al. "Sugarcane Molasses – A Potential Dietary Supplement in the Management of Iron Deficiency Anemia." Journal of Dietary Supplements, 14:5, 589-598, DOI: 10.1080/19390211.2016.1269145, 26 Jan. 2017

Marengo, Katherine. "Evidence-Based Benefits of Apple Cider Vinegar and How to Use It." Medical News Today, MediLexicon International. *https://www.medicalnewstoday.com/articles/323721#takeaway*

Morgan, Joanna and Mosawy, Sapha. "The Potential of Apple Cider Vinegar in the Management of Type 2 Diabetes." (2016).

Newman, Tim. "High Blood Pressure: Sodium May Not Be the Culprit." Medical News Today, MediLexicon International. *https://www.medicalnewstoday.com/articles/317099*

Salehi, Bahare, et al. "Resveratrol: A Double-Edged Sword in Health Benefits." Biomedicines, U.S. National Library of Medicine, 9 Sept. 2018. *https://www.ncbi.nlm.nih.gov/pmc/articles/PMC6164842*

ScienceDaily. "Low-Sodium Diet Might Not Lower Blood Pressure." ScienceDaily, 25 Apr. 2017. *https://www.sciencedaily.com/releases/2017/04/170425124909.htm*

Tiralongo, Evelin, et al. "Elderberry Supplementation Reduces Cold Duration and Symptoms in Air-Travellers: A Randomized, Double-Blind Placebo-Controlled Clinical Trial." Nutrients, U.S. National Library of Medicine, 24 Mar. 2016. *https://www.ncbi.nlm.nih.gov/pmc/articles/PMC4848651/*

Valli, Veronica et al. "Sugar Cane and Sugar Beet Molasses Alternatives to Refined Sugars." ACS Publications: Chemistry Journals, Books, and References Published. J. Agri. Food Chem, 26 Dec. 2012, *https://pubs.acs.org/doi/abs/10.1021/jf304416d*

Chapter 23: Elimination

Cleveland Clinic. "What Your Poop Type and Color Says about You." Cleveland Clinic, 12 Dec. 2022. *https://health.clevelandclinic.org/healthy-poop-shape-type-color*

Malone, Jordan, et al. "Physiology, Gastrocolic Reflex." Statpearls - NCBI Bookshelf. *https://www.ncbi.nlm.nih.gov/books/NBK549888*

ScienceDaily. "A Sauna Session Is Just as Exhausting as Moderate Exercise, Study Finds." ScienceDaily, 12 June 2019. *https://www.sciencedaily.com/releases/2019/06/190612093900.htm*

Chapter 24: Exercise (Mindful Movement)

Breus, Michael. "Chronotypes." The Sleep Doctor, 13 Dec. 2022. *https://thesleepdoctor.com/how-sleep-works/chronotypes*

Hong, A Ram, and Kim, Sang Wan. "Effects of Resistance Exercise on Bone Health." Endocrinology and Metabolism (Seoul, Korea), U.S. National Library of Medicine, Dec. 2018. *https://www.ncbi.nlm.nih.gov/pmc/articles/PMC6279907*

Law, TD; Clark, LA; Clark, BC. "Resistance Exercise to Prevent and Manage Sarcopenia and Dynapenia." Annu Rev Gerontol Geriatr.

2016;36(1):205-228. doi: 10.1891/0198-8794.36.205. PMID: 27134329; PMCID: PMC4849483

Weir, Kirsten. "Nurtured by Nature." Monitor on Psychology, American Psychological Association. *https://www.apa.org/monitor/2020/04/ nurtured-nature*

White, Mathew P., et al. "Spending at Least 120 Minutes a Week in Nature Is Associated with Good Health and Wellbeing." Nature News, Nature Publishing Group, 13 June 2019. *https://www.nature.com/articles/ s41598-019-44097-3*

Chapter 25: Energy Drainers

NIEHS. "Bisphenol A (BPA)." National Institute of Environmental Health Sciences, U.S. Department of Health and Human Services. *https://www. niehs.nih.gov/health/topics/agents/sya-bpa/index.cfm*

NIEHS. "Cell Phone Radio Frequency Radiation." National Institute of Environmental Health Sciences, U.S. Department of Health and Human Services. *https://ntp.niehs.nih.gov/whatwestudy/topics/cellphones*

NIEHS. "Electric & Magnetic Fields." National Institute of Environmental Health Sciences, U.S. Department of Health and Human Services. *https:// www.niehs.nih.gov/health/topics/agents/emf/index.cfm*

Pang, Qihua, et al. "Neurotoxicity of BPA, BPS, and BPB for the Hippocampal Cell Line (HT-22): An Implication for the Replacement of BPA in Plastics." Chemosphere, U.S. National Library of Medicine. *https://pubmed.ncbi.nlm.nih.gov/30953899/#:~:text=Bisphenol percent20A percent20(BPA) percent2C percent20a,and percent20bisphenol percent20B percent20(BPB)*

Nielsen. "Time Flies: U.S. Adults Now Spend Nearly Half a Day Interacting with Media." Nielsen, 21 July 2022. *https://www.nielsen.com/insights/2018/ time-flies-us-adults-now-spend-nearly-half-a-day-interacting-with-media/#:~:- text=According percent20to percent20the percent20first percent2Dquarter,or percent20generally percent20interacting percent20with percent20media*

Williams, Trevicia. "An Unsuspecting Link to Sleep Deprivation and Stress." Psychology Today, Sussex Publishers. *https://www.psychologytoday. com/us/blog/strong-lives/202205/unsuspecting-link-sleep-deprivation-and-stress*

Chapter 26: Energy Enhancers

Drake, Christopher, et al. "Caffeine Effects on Sleep Taken 0, 3, or 6 Hours before Going to Bed." Journal of Clinical Sleep Medicine : JCSM : Official Publication of the American Academy of Sleep Medicine, U.S. National Library of Medicine, 15 Nov. 2013. *https://www.ncbi.nlm.nih.gov/pmc/articles/ PMC3805807/#:~:text=Conclusion percent3A,6 percent20hours percent20prior percent20to percent20bedtime*

Schmid, Sebastian, et al. "A Single Night of Sleep Deprivation Increases Ghrelin Levels and Feelings of Hunger in Normal-Weight Healthy Men." Journal of Sleep Research, U.S. National Library of Medicine. *https:// pubmed.ncbi.nlm.nih.gov/18564298/*

Chapter 27: Become Your FINE Self

Morris, ZS et al. "The Answer is 17 Years, What is the Question: Understanding Time Lags in Translational Research." Journal of the Royal Society of Medicine. *https://www.ncbi.nlm.nih.gov/pmc/articles/ PMC3241518/#:~:text=It percent20is percent20frequently percent20stated percent20that,evidence percent20to percent20reach percent20clinical percent20practice.*

INDEX

B

C

www.ingramcontent.com/pod-product-compliance
Lightning Source LLC
Chambersburg PA
CBHW032049020426
42335CB00011B/260